My Open Heart Surgery

Loury N. Cortez

and

The Day of
My Aneurysm

Are you a walking time bomb?

Copyright © Loury N. Cortez 2015
Illustrations copyright © Loury N. Cortez 2014, J.B Talagtag 2014, Krystina Bogus 2014
Photographs © Loury N. Cortez 2015
Cover design and book layout: Nettie O'Connell - www.nettieodesign.com
Publisher/Imprint: Loury N. Cortez – CN1798943

National Library of Australia Cataloguing-in-Publication entry
Creator: Cortez, Loury N., author.
Title: My open heart surgery and the day of my aneurysm / Loury N. Cortez
ISBN: 9780646953960 (paperback)
Notes: Includes bibliographical references.
Subjects: Cortez, Loury N.
        1. Heart–Surgery–Patients–Australia–Biography
        2. Abdominal aneurysm–Australia
        3. Aortic aneurysms–Australia
Dewey Number: 617.412092

Bibliography
Cortez, Loury N.
Heart/Abdominal Aortic Aneurysm-Surgery-Patients- Volunteer-Australia-Biography

This book is for information and educational purposes only, it does not replace, nor
should it be considered and alternative to, medical advice. In case of illness or injury,
you should consult your doctor.

To my wife Nela and son Darren
and
my brother Peter and sisters Patricia, Juanita and Maree

Life is either a daring adventure,
or
Nothing.
Helen Keller

Don't stress and worry
about things
that you cannot control.
Unknown

Be a warrior
Get your One Point
and
Extend your Ki.
Loury N. Cortez

CONTENTS

BOOK ONE
My Open Heart Surgery

BOOK TWO
The Day of My Aneurysm

ABOUT THE AUTHOR

Born Loreto Lawrence Noble Cortez in 1937, Loury's mother was Australian; his father was from the Philippines. Loury attended High School in Manila in the early 1950s and returned to Melbourne in 1954 to become an Aircraft Mechanic.

He went to Papua New Guinea (PNG) in the sixties for a period of six years but stayed for 25 years. He was a Community Primary School Head Teacher; a Shipping Manager for San Miguel and Swan Brewery. OIC Physical Training Wing at the Bomana Police College where he taught self-defence (Arnis-Philippine Stick Fighting) and weapons training. In the 1980s he was Chief of Security for the PNG National Parliament and worked for the Department of the Prime Minister, as Assistant Secretary Building and Security Services.

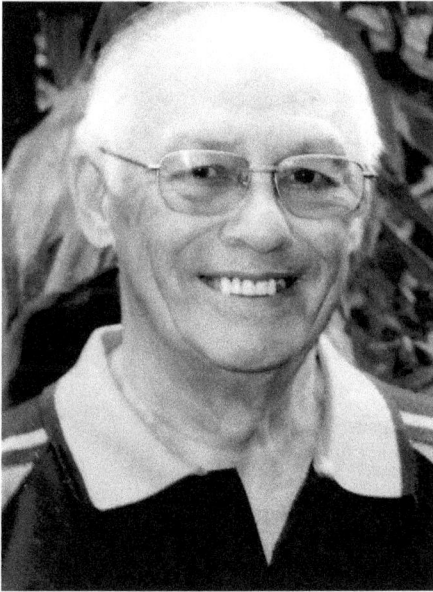

In the mid 1970s he became the PNG National Basketball Coach. He coached both men and women at junior and senior level in Port Moresby, Cairns and Melbourne; in the late 1970s he was the Secretary General of the PNG Sports Federation that encompassed the Olympics, Commonwealth and South Pacific Games Committees; he was a member of the PNG National Sports Council, and a director of the PNG Sports Aid foundation. Loury was also involved in various other sports.

He is married to Nela of 47 years and together with their son Darren they live in Cairns, Queensland, Australia.

Loury N. Cortez

FOREWORD

I have been a cardiac surgeon for over 20 years. We are trained to recognize all potential complications in cardiac Surgery. We were never taught to enter the "Sphere" of patient's experience following their surgery. This is a fascinating account of a patient's journey going through open heart operation. It is a very descriptive account from the initial consultation right through the recovery phase following his surgery. As surgeons we often took things for granted and only looked at the patient's data and test results. Based on these, we assume the patients are doing alright. This manuscript gave me an insight of the patient's experience and taught me to spend more time in our ward rounds instead of running through all the figures and not listening to patients.

Assoc. Prof Robert Tam
Director, Cardiothoracic Surgery
The Townsville Hospital
P.O.Box 670
Townsville Qld 4810

PRELUDE

Loury Cortez has done a fine job in writing about his experiences as a cardiac patient both at Cairns Base Hospital and Townsville Hospital. It has been very interesting to read about his journey through the eyes of a patient which is indeed a very different insight than that of hospital staff who encounter these events on a daily basis. I am sure that patients who have been newly diagnosed with a cardiac condition will learn from Loury's experiences and patients who already had similar experiences will relate to his amusing stories. This is a true testament to the vital work that our Cardiac Rehab team does at Cairns Base Hospital, including the essential volunteers, and it is pleasing to have a patient acknowledge these services.

Wishing all patients as successful a recovery as Loury's...

Dr V.R. Prasad Challa
Director of Cardiology
Cairns Base Hospital

PRELUDE

Heart disease is the most prevalent disease affecting our nation today, robbing us of one of our precious Australians every 22 minutes. With statistics like that there is no doubt that most Australians will be touched by the effects of heart disease, whether it is a loved one or them self.

Advances in Cardiology have provided safe and effective treatment options for heart disease saving numerous lives every day. Fortunately we are able to access highly effective cardiac medications, and procedures such as Angioplasty and stenting and cardiac surgery in the form of "bypass" surgery.

Those given the news that they require cardiac surgery are often overwhelmed, anxious, confused and angry. Cardiac educators spend a great deal of time with the patient and their family discussing the surgery, reassuring through education and support. Although effective, there is nothing more valuable in this situation as firsthand experience, a person who has been through the procedure and come out the other side stronger and healthier than before to share their experiences.

Loury Cortez has travelled this rocky road of cardiac surgery, not only requiring bypass surgery but valve replacement to fix a poorly functioning valve. Loury's book recalls the journey from diagnosis to surgery and recovery in cardiac rehabilitation. His story is told through the eyes of a positive and inspirational man who has the ability to make the most of each of life's experiences, even being able to see the funny side of Cardiac Surgery.

Although seemingly impossible, positivity at this time is instrumental in expediting recovery. Loury's positive outlook allowed him to overcome the challenges he had post-surgery and saw him excel in Cardiac Rehabilitation and go on to be an invaluable volunteer in the Cairns Base Hospital Cardiac Rehabilitation program. Each day he inspires the patients and staff with his optimistic and enthusiastic nature and unique sense of humour.

If you or your loved one is preparing for cardiac surgery or you are reading this book out of general interest, take inspiration from Loury's story. Any of life's journeys will be so much less troublesome if faced with insight, a sense of humour and a positive attitude.

Mandi Pashley
Cardiac Rehab Coordinator

ACKNOWLEDGEMENTS

I would like to thank the following people and organizations for their kindness in offering their expertise and information in the writing of both my journeys.

Dr Robert Tam MBBS, FRACS, FRAC (CT) Director, Cardiothoracic Surgery, Townsville Hospital and his team of Dr Rajiv and Dr Alveska, what can I say, you were there for me and opened the alien writer that lurked within this human body. Dr V. 'Prasad' Challa, Director of Cardiology, Cairns Base Hospital who assessed my Coronary Angiogram, resulting in the need for an aortic valve replacement and a triple by-pass graft that hit me for a six! Dr Neil Brodie MB.B.S. has been our GP for the last 22 years, and Dr Derrick Coetzee MBChB. FRACGP, of South Care Medical Centre, Woree.

To Mandi Pashley, Cardiac Coordinator Nurse CBH, thank you for your helpful hints, insights and for vetting the medical side of the story, an angel who helped my recovery. My thanks also to Cardiac Nurses Brenda Joyce-Dunn, Jacqueline Cairns, Anita Basu, Yvonne Hodder, Dawn Newman, Angie Sutcliffe, Cheryl Hastie, Midge Balodis Cardiac Nurse Manager and Kylie Sommerville our Cardiac rehab physiotherapist. To all the staff of the Cairns Base Hospital (CBH) and the Townsville Hospital, especially the Coronary Cardiac Unit and Med 3 without whose dedication, people like me would not have benefited from your caring nature.

That marvelous group of cardiac rehabilitation volunteers, the purple people eaters of Graham Cox (dec.) Tom Spearman (dec.) Glen Hannaford (dec.) Nick Stocker, Anne Hewitt, Brian Ball, Les McLaren, Ann Mather and Karen Chapman who have given their time to ensure that my rehabilitation and recovery was a success. What a team! What a family! FNQ Hospital Foundation their value to the volunteers and the community goes without saying, fantastic! My thanks to the men and women of the Queensland Ambulance Service their dedication is well above the call of duty. Go the Ambos! Without them patients would be left in the wilderness.

The Heart Foundation of Australia for all the information and literature that is supplied to help provide the patient with a better understanding of their health problems. To Pfizer Australia Pty Limited for all the information, literature about lowering one's cholesterol towards having a healthy lifestyle. My thanks to the staff of the Westcourt

Community Health and Support Services, Queensland Health.

What can I say, but this is a friendship of a lifetime, my thanks to Sue and Gary Schofield, Marietta Percali and daughter Sharleen. To the Philippine connection, my sister-in-law Dr Lucita P. Zamora and my niece, Dr Aisa R. Presas, your personal information helped me understand the possible ramifications of my operation.

To my gallant proofreaders my appreciation and thanks to Gary Schofield, John Nash, Lloyd Binion, Ron Clarke, Ngaire Tagney for doing such a sterling job. From Manila, Philippines J.B.Talatag who produced the caricatures. Nettie O'Connell of nettieodesign.com for the book design and layout, and contributors Mandi Pashely and Nela P. Cortez. To my son Darren, what more can I ask, you were there for me.

Last and not least to my wife, Nela P. Cortez, who was my carer and confidant, you are my shining light.

INTRODUCTION

You're feeling low, tormented by hundreds of 'what ifs', you're pussyfooting around the house and with each step your heart beat is magnified, you are terrified, you want to do things, but diligently you follow the instructions given to you after your open heart surgery. Don't lift more than 5kgs in the first six weeks; avoid strenuous movements for three months. You panic when faced with a few setbacks, one step forward and three steps back.

You enter the cardiac rehabilitation program, distressed, your mind asks, "What's the use? What can it do to reduce my future plumbing and pumping situations?" It's maddening but what can it do to free my mind from all the 'what ifs'. Apprehension is washed away as my survival instinct kicks in and I enter the realms of learning a new lifestyle.

My Open Heart Surgery

Loury N. Cortez

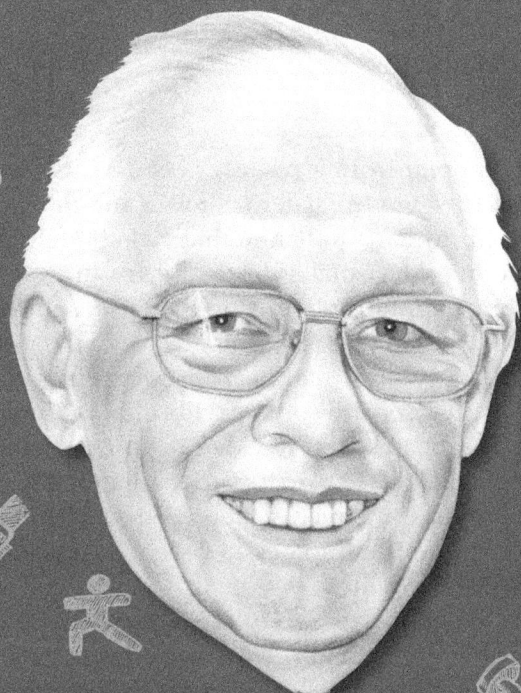

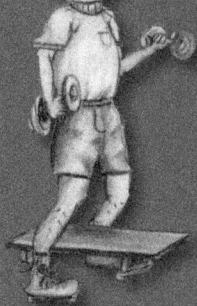

action rehab

GYM

WORK OUT

DIET

BMI

Chapter 1
How it Began

I forced my leaden eyes to open from a restless sleep. Wearily I sat on the bed for several minutes then got up, had my shower and my usual shave. But the magical splash of my Paco Rabanne that Nela bought me at Christmas did little to give me that usual sparkle and freshness of a clean shaven face. Combing my hair, I felt slightly off colour despite the reflection of the clear blue skies and the trees off the surface of the pool.

It was a day in December 2006, and I had been showing symptoms of tiredness and lethargy, and a few seconds of heart fibrillation the day before. Although showing no real concern, I decided to visit my GP Dr Neil Brodie, South Care Medical Centre, Woree. Unfortunately for me he had left with his family to go on Christmas vacation. Lucky him! Me? My wife Nela had taken a trip to the Philippines to visit her family and here I was home alone with our dog 'Bella.'

However, I was able to get an appointment with Dr Derrick Coetzee, who upon hearing of my problem attached his trusty stethoscope and detected a systolic murmur in my heart. He decided that I needed to go for a blood test, chest x-ray and an echocardiographic examination.

Several weeks later and Swish! Swish! Nothing but a heartbeat, and the results of the echocardiogram (ECG) examination indicated to Dr Coetzee that I should be checked out by a specialist. A referral was made at the Cairns Base Hospital. Initially I met with an attending cardiac doctor who conferred with Dr V 'Prasad' Challa, the Director of the Cardiac Investigations Unit concerning the echo examination. I was told via a sketch on a pad that the blood flow pressure in the aortic valve area was slightly high. Although there was no cause for alarm at this stage, it was decided that I should have annual check-ups and that I should now include 30 minute walks as part of my daily exercise regimen, i.e. swimming, gardening etc. However, 2006 rolled into 2007 and flew into 2008. The results of these annual checkups were within the prescribed pressure limits and there was no cause for concern or was there?

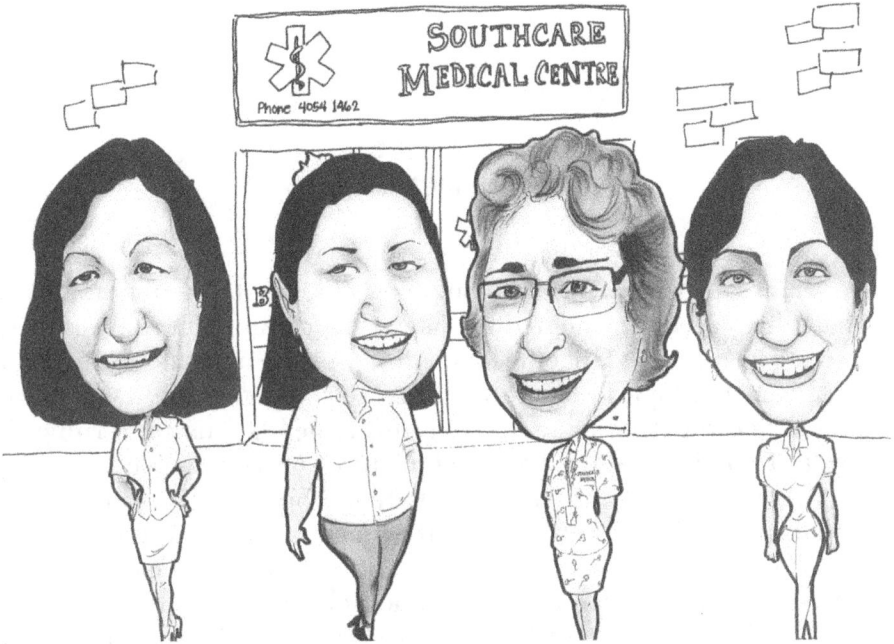

Sue   Kylie   Helen   Sandy

Chapter 2
Annual Check-up

Things to Come. Prior to my November, 2008 appointment, Dr Challa had already examined my latest echocardiogram results. At our meeting he explained that the blood flow pressure from the aortic region had reached a high level and that a coronary angiogram was required to ascertain the problem and make recommendations concerning the results. I wondered at the time if a puncture kit was available!

Are you ready for it? Heart valves are like one-way doors that control the direction of blood flow between the four chambers of the heart. In my case, the symptoms indicated that the aortic valve was damaged and was *not closing properly*; this allowed blood to flow back into the left ventricle chamber and not into the blood vessels supplying the rest of my body. This defect is called an incompetent or regurgitant valve. On the other hand, a damaged valve which limits forward blood flow by *not opening properly* is called a stenotic valve. Like a door opening and closing. Did that make sense?

My first question was, "When will the angiogram take place?" Dr Challa advised that it would take place in the New Year as the present schedules were completely full. I replied, "That's alright as long as it is not until after March, 2009 as my family and I have booked our vacation trip to the Philippines during March and April."

This was my major concern as my son Darren and his friend Danni were really looking forward to the trip and to have it canceled at this stage would be heart-breaking. Rather than focusing on the pending procedure, I decided to follow up with a letter to Dr Challa concerning the above and asked him to consider this when making his deliberations about a possible operation.

To no avail! I was offered a coronary angiogram appointment courtesy of the Cardiac Investigations Unit.

What is it? An electrocardiogram (ECG) is a medical test that detects cardiac (heart) abnormalities by measuring the electrical activity generated by the heart as it contracts. An ECG is completely painless and non-invasive as the skin is in no way penetrated.

An electrocardiogram is done to:

- Check the heart's electrical activity
- Find the cause of unexplained *chest pain*, which could be caused by *heart attack*, inflammation of the sac surrounding the heart *(pericarditis)*, or *angina*.
- Find the causes of symptoms of *heart disease*, such as shortness of breath, *dizziness*, *fainting*, or rapid, irregular heartbeats (palpitations).
- Find out if the walls of the heart chambers are too thick (hypertrophied).
- Check how well medicines are working and whether they are causing side effects that affect the heart.
- Check how well mechanical devices that are implanted in the heart, such as *pacemakers*, are working to control a normal heartbeat.
- Check the health of the heart when other diseases or conditions are present, such as *high blood pressure*, *high cholesterol*, cigarette *smoking*, *diabetes*.

(WebMedical Reference from Healthwise 11 September, 2012)

Chapter 3
Coronary Angiogram

Come Off It! Aortic valve… triple by-pass! Who me? No way! I walked into the Cairns Base Hospital that Monday, physically fit, no indications of dizziness, no pain, blood pressure was slightly high, no shortage of breath but I came out of the hospital bodily sick!

Out of the blue – I was booked to go for my coronary angiogram on 9th December 2008; of course the mind begins to play tricks and all sorts of things revolve about the outcome. However, I take time to do my deep breathing exercise and my philosophy of, *why stress out if I'm not in control,* my mind clears and I relax. I'll leave it to the experts!

A blood test, a chest X-ray and an ECG were done a few days prior to the angiogram test. Before leaving home, I had a triclosan (antiseptic wash) shower, dressed and then drove the 15 minutes to the Cairns Base Hospital.

Ironically, I had been reading a fictional novel several weeks earlier about a husband and wife who were both coroners. The husband had broken his leg and was all set for an operation at a particular hospital that his wife was investigating. She had advised the husband not to go for the operation at the hospital because of several unexplained deaths caused by golden staph infections, but in reply, he said "Don't worry! For the past several weeks I've been washing myself thoroughly with a good, antibacterial wash." This information began to play on my mind so I went out and bought some Sapoderm antibacterial soap which I used constantly prior to the cardio angiogram test and right up to my forthcoming operation.

Taking the elevator to the 3rd Floor 'B' Block, I waited until I was called and taken into the CIU Ward. Six patients, and I was the first cab off the rank - an early start, a quick change into hospital pj's, onto the bed, the nurse takes my pulse, respirations, blood pressure, the hair on my right wrist is shaved for the wrist (radial) approach. A cannula is placed into my arm and I receive a pre-medication tablet that makes me drowsy but I'm still aware of what was happening in the ward.

After all this preparation I'm wheeled into an elevator and taken on a sightseeing tour to the Medical Imaging Department. I wait in the corridor watching the doctors, nurses and orderlies flashing pass and contemplate what they would look like in brightly, coloured uniforms that would depict life for the patient, but more importantly they would be easily identifiable not only to the patients but also the public. Gazing at the ceiling, walls and charts that are part of the hospital décor, I envisage delightful art work showing our Reef and Rain Forest.

Finally the wait is over; I'm taken into the operating Theatre. The nurses are wearing gowns and masks to protect me from any infection, they ask me to lie on the procedural table then the ECG electrodes are attached to my chest to monitor the functions of my heart. Sterile drapes are placed over me like a tablecloth; was this the last supper, I reflect! There is constant chatter between the nurses and the doctor, then the wait is over as Dr Challa, dressed in blue, starts his preparation for the procedure.

My wrist (radial approach) is cleaned with the orange red Betadine antiseptic. It is a relaxed atmosphere, as Dr Challa continues to converse with the nurses, he tells me that I can watch the procedure on the closed circuit TV. He then injects a local anaesthetic to numb the area. Then begins the cardio angiogram procedure by inserting a plastic tube into the blood vessel where-in the image-intensifier (camera) is able to track the movement of the tube on its journey to my heart.

I'm amazed at the technology and struggle to watch all of it on the TV screen. At times I feel like Indianna Jones in the "Raiders of the Lost Ark" as the image intensifier moves to and fro, sometimes hovering, as it lowers ever-so-close to my chest, my neck strains to catch a glimpse of what is happening on the TV but to no avail. Sometimes I'm asked to cough or do certain things and suddenly I experience a warm, flush feeling throughout my body, a dye has been injected into me and this helps Dr Challa in monitoring the procedure.

Finally the procedure is completed and I'm wheeled back to the Cardiac Investigation Unit (CIU) for my recovery and to await the verdict.

Since I had the radial approach, the catheter is removed and I had to stay in the CIU for 90 minutes, but my pulse and blood pressure is monitored on a regular basis. In the meantime, the puncture site had to be frequently checked to ensure that there was no excessive bleeding or swelling. To guarantee that there was a good circulation of blood either my hand or foot was assessed for a strong pulse via the artery.

In time the nurse has asked me to change into my day clothes and to vacate the bed for a more comfortable, recliner chair. I'm famished and mention this to the nurse, who like a magician provides me with a sandwich and a drink.

I watch the proceedings in the ward with interest and liken it to a chess game; as patients are moved in and out of the ward for their turn in the theatre under the steady hands of the light, fingered Challa. I'm sure in his younger days he would have been a good spin bowler as he really enjoys his cricket.

The last patient has returned to the ward, and about 1:30pm Dr Challa walks triumphantly into the ward with his ever, gleaming smile, indicating another successful day for him and his team, and to pass on his findings to us. For each of us the waiting is over.

It is my turn, "Loury you will need an aortic valve replacement," he said. Then he uttered, "You will also need a triple By-pass as one artery is 90% closed and the other two are about 70% closed". My mouth drops and I look at him amazement and said, "But my cholesterol has always being 2.5 to 3.0 and I've had no symptoms whatsoever and now I need a triple by-pass!" I had assumed that when my cholesterol had a low reading, then my arteries were ok.' Dr Challa said, "There are other types of cholesterol that can trigger the problem." In reply, I said, "I cannot recall any doctor telling me about the bad cholesterol. I wish I had more knowledge about those other causes, but I am glad the procedure was successful."

Speaking to his assistant, Dr Challa said, "Loury will need 80mg of Atorvastatin to be included with his current medication and the GTN spray, and we will also schedule an appointment with the Cardiothoracic Surgery Case Coordinator, who will contact you concerning other requirements that will be needed." He wishes me luck and walks towards another patient.

Later I discover that there is, the good guy, HDL Cholesterol that doesn't get deposited in the arteries; the bad guy LDL Cholesterol that causes fatty deposits in the lining of the arteries which can cause your risk of heart attack; the Ugly guy the Triglyceride (TG) high levels often mean HDL is too low, combining the high TG + LDL can further increase your risk of heart disease. (Pocket Guide to Cholesterol lowering 'Lipitor' atorvastatin calcium) Well that certainly got your attention and are you more confused than me? You will be able to read more towards the end of the book.

I was not unduly worried about the turn of events, and again my deep breathing exercises and the response to stress was, *if I'm not in control I won't stress out*. My immediate thought was that our vacation will have to be cancelled and put on hold till the end of next year. Here I was thinking that I might be lucky to have the operation postponed, what wishful thinking.

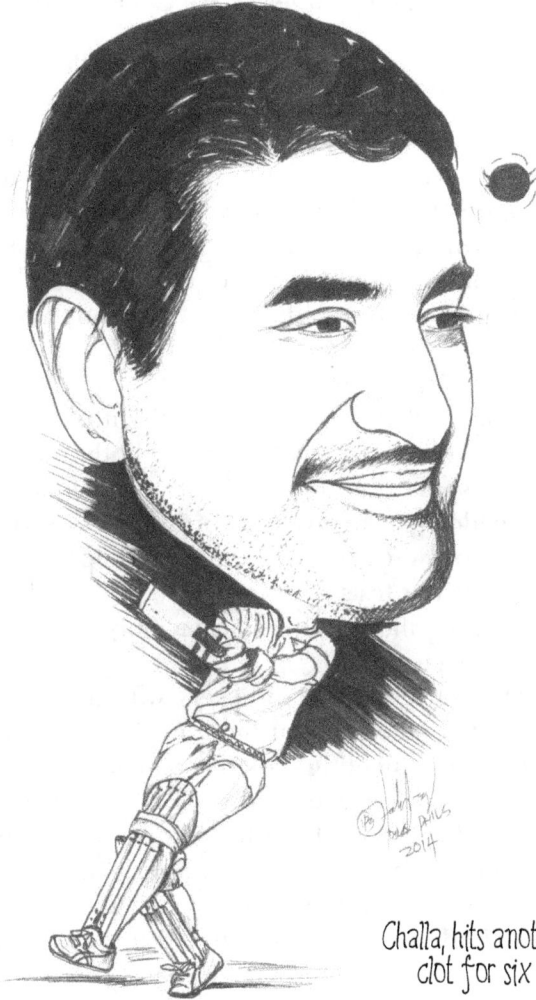

Challa, hits another
clot for six

Chapter 4
Cardiothoracic Surgery Case Coordinator

Information Time. The subsequent outcome of the Coronary Angiogram test resulted in Dr Challa recommending a referral to the cardiothoracic surgeons for consideration in regards to a severe aortic regurgitation (Grade IV) replacement and a triple disease (RCA, LCx and CAD) via a coronary artery bypass graft (CABG) surgery. Highly technical information, but confusing to us mere mortals.

Wouldn't it be great if they said, 'you have a puncture that has to be repaired with a new valve and we are going to take tubes from your leg and join them up in your heart?'

On 13th January 2009, enters the delightful, friendly, blonde Cheryl Hastie, the clinical nurse and the Cardiothoracic Surgery Case Coordinator. Cheryl spoke about her role as a coordinator and what was to occur. She proceeded to take my blood pressure, asked questions about my current medications etc., then gave me the appropriate paperwork for me to undergo further tests that needed to be completed before our meeting with the Townsville hospital Cardiac Surgeon, Dr Tam that was scheduled for 16 February 2009.

Calling for an archaeological discovery within my human body, a blood test, a chest x-ray, an electrocardiogram (ECG) and a dental check were required before the meeting took place in February.

My dental check took place at the CBH Dental Clinic with the inevitable probing of gums and teeth. X-Rays were taken and it was decided that a tooth connected to my bridge had to be extracted. Ironically, a year previously, it was a same tooth that met the skills of a dentist and an Orthodontist but it continued to decay, after numerous outings. I should have had it removed then and there as it would have saved me heaps of dollars.

Before any dental work was carried out, it was essential for me to take in 2g of Amoxycillin, a prophylactic antibiotic to ensure that there was no infection in the system when I had to undergo surgery. I certainly did not want any aliens playing around my open chest! However, the dentist needed to query the actual dosage as it seemed a lot.

The extraction took place on 22 January and prior to the procedure the dentist said, 'I've rechecked the X-ray and have concluded that another tooth located at the rear of the mouth is not required and should also be removed. The dentist advised that she would be very careful in the extraction and would try to ensure that the bridge did not suffer any damage during the procedure otherwise I would need a new bridge.

Before starting she gave me the 2g Amoxycillin tablet, I looked at it and said, 'You must be joking!' The tablet was the size of a dinner plate but I forced it down with large quantities of water and then had to wait an hour for it to take effect.

Back into the chair for the extraction to take place. A deadening agent, a few stinging jabs from the needle and I felt like Louis Armstrong as my mouth was swollen and then with the pliers, a tight grip and *Viola!* The teeth are out. I now have a nice gap and my smile could now be likened to Batman's Cave.

Weeks later I was called into the clinic to have a prosthesis tooth inserted in the gap, of course, the dentist told me "This was a temporary measure but it was good for my smile especially if I had photos taken at a wedding or a party."

Chapter 5
Dr Robert Tam

Decision Time. It is 16 February 2009 and Nela and I take the elevator to the 6th Floor of Block B at the CBH and present myself and paperwork to the receptionist at the Cardiac Thoracic Clinic.

I have read all the available literature given to me and downloaded some information from the Internet that helps towards making the right decision concerning the type of valve to be used i.e. the mechanical valve or the tissue (biological) valve. However, I needed to ask further questions of Dr Tam about them and the medications that I would need to take after the operation.

I finally meet with Dr Robert Tam. He is a Malaysian-Australian, quiet, unassuming. During the interview he asks the inevitable health questions and asks several times my reason for seeing him. I realize that this is necessary for the patient and the doctor to verify quite clearly what is to occur in the very near future.

One question I ask is, "If you are going to do two operations will it take six hours or longer as the information infers that each operation will take about three hours each?" Dr Tam smiled and said; "No!" It will be about three hours as the other team will be removing the veins from your leg at the same time as I am operating on your heart."

Dr Tam has inserted the DVD of my electrocardiogram results and finally I get to see my heart in action as during the ECG I hear the swishing sounds. Dr Tam explains to Nela and me where the problems lie and what he intends to do during the operation. He said, "I will cut down the midline of your chest, through the breastbone, to reach your heart. During surgery your body will be kept cool to protect the vital organs by slowing down their working rate so that they need less oxygen. A heart-lung machine takes over the function of your heart and lungs."

"Thank God I am an avid fan of RPA (Royal Prince Alfred) TV program! I've seen it before and now it's going to happen to me!" I muse and think to myself, *I hope they have quiet music I don't want them doing a jive whilst the cutting procedure takes place, a nice straight cut will be fine.*

I asked, "Will I need a blood transfusion?" In reply, he said, "If there is a need for a blood transfusion, rest easy as all blood products used for the transfusion in Australia are strictly screened to protect patients against viruses that can cause hepatitis and AIDS."

So it is decision time, "What valve replacement do you want?" Dr Tam asks me as he picks up his pen. I decided to have the mechanical valve because they last longer but I still have some reservations concerning possible blood clots and the warfarin anti-coagulant medication for life! Dr Tam makes note of this all important decision.

Dr Tam advises that I will be placed on the waiting list for a heart valve replacement and a triple bypass graft at the Townsville Hospital. This could take up to eight weeks or more! He wishes me well as we shake hands and Nela and I leave the interview room.

After leaving Dr Tam we receive further information from Cheryl Hastie, in regards to travel, accommodation. She provides us with a travel voucher which we take to the travel department CBH on the ground floor. We are told that the voucher will be processed once they have the actual surgery date.

Well the die is cast, and the holiday trip we have been looking forward to all year, to the Philippines, will be cancelled. Unfortunately, the paid holiday airfares package and accommodation to a Manila beach resort for us and some of our family members has been lost! "What will be? Will be." But I am not dispirited. Now onto the next step.

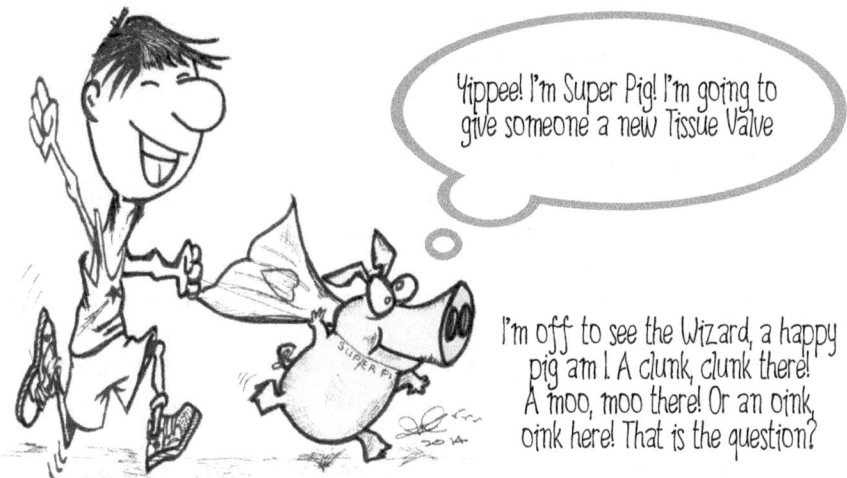

Chapter 6
Time to Tell Relations and Friends

Caring Friends. I fleetingly ruminate about telling my relations and our friends about my problem! Do I get them involved? Do they need to know? What will they say? Will it be out of self-pity or will they talk about distant relations who have had the same problem and the pain that was involved?

Will they try to tell me what to do, to prepare for an unseen battle that may never occur? While all these thoughts twirl about my mind like zephyrs across the desert sands, I realize that I am making mountains out of molehills and whatever happens, these are my caring friends.

I rang my sisters, Pat, Juanita, Maree and my brother Peter and share the news of my pending surgery. Immediately they all wanted to come to be with me. I thank them for their love and support and mention to them that I have yet to have the operation. However, their insistence caused me to say, "Let's wait until after the op and to see how well I am coping." I appreciated their help, but it was a case of not putting undue stress on us, especially Nela who would be my carer during the months ahead.

Having read all the literature that was given to me, I noted that I would need my own space, rest and the time to regain my energy and physical being for me to get back into a recovery mode.

Then a phone call in early February caused a small problem. It was from Nela's cousin Vicky from the Philippines. She and her American husband Steve had arrived in Melbourne in January for a holiday to visit Vicky's son Michael.

Vicky said, "Steve and I are planning to visit you for a few days and we will come up by train." I spoke to them and told them of the situation and that we were waiting for the call to travel to Townsville for me to undergo the surgery. Again, not wanting to hurt their feelings, I had to thank them for their support, but it would not be possible as we really did not want to look after visitors when we had numerous other things to consider. They understood, however, their numerous phone calls over several weeks and wanting to know if I had the op and when they could come to Cairns was gratifying.

Our house is often likened to a hotel and it was not in my character to refuse our visitors a big welcome, unfortunately this was one case where I had to stand firm! Was this a sign of stress?

I have yet to tell my Aunt Rose and my cousins in Seattle USA as I did not want them to unduly worry—especially my aunt who is 83 years old and at 72 I'm her brother's son and a favourite nephew.

Que Sera, Sera! It's the last week in March and the phone ring. I answer it wondering if this was the call-up. "Hi, Loury it's Cousin Linda." "Well this is a pleasant surprise what's up?" I said. In reply she asks if I have a pencil and paper. "Yes" I said, thinking that she wanted me to buy her something from Cairns. Linda replied laughing, "Pick me up on 4th April; I'll be with you for a month." She proceeded to give me her Flight details and told me that she had a great promotional deal from the USA to fly to Australia and it was too good to pass up. Oh! "By the way have you had your operation?" She asked. I was completely flabbergasted and explained the situation and that I was still waiting for a call from the Townsville Hospital.

Who let the cat out of the bag, I asked myself! Here I am telling people not to come and, low and behold my American cousin from Seattle is flying into Cairns, I feel like a heel! It was surely a case of 'déjà vu.' It was time to break the news to the rest of the family in Manila.

We contact Nela's sister Lucy to tell her about the pending operation and that our trip to Manila has now been cancelled. She was disappointed and the rest of the family would also have the same feelings. Being a doctor, Lucy thoroughly understood our situation and advised us not to try and change things in order to make the trip. She said, "You have better medical facilities in Australia and the whole family would be stressed out watching over you and hoping that nothing occurs in the form of a stroke or heart attack whilst in the Philippines." I replied, *Rest assured I would not put you through that kind of stress.*

We contact Franz and Eva in the Tablelands; Ian and Gloria at Mareeba; Lex and Margaret McCreath at Ravenshoe. They could not get over the idea that I needed an operation as their comments were, "He's always happy, smiling and has partially laid 120 pavers on the 4 square meters of crusher dust laid on the side pathway. He's fit and shows good health; there must be some mistake?" "How can he be sick?" There lurks the question?

Being good friends, they wish me a successful operation when it comes to fruition and to contact them for any reason, if I need help. How long I have to wait is the unknown target.

Chapter 7
The Waiting Period

Not Yet! *What is the relevance of all this writing*, I muse as I put pen to paper?

Strong emotions sometimes cloud our judgments, our thoughts and we need to be fully motivated not to fall into the trap of *why me?* However, at the end of the day we all deal with things in our own way. This was my way!

Well, following my meeting with Dr Tam in February, I realized that after a few weeks, I had unconsciously been pussy-footing around, taking it easy rather than doing the things that needed to be done. I had to get back on track! Rather than wait with bated breath for that all important phone call to tell us to pack our bags, and to make our way to Townsville Hospital. But not yet.

It was time for a change so I stepped up my exercises and with Cousin Linda arriving on the 4th April I needed to spend some time writing out an itinerary, as to what we will do and see, so that she can really appreciate our Paradise in Cairns.

I celebrated my 72nd birthday on 11 April 2009 and we were invited to lunch with Eva and Franz Scholl at Atherton. Clear blue skies makes for a good days drive up the Kuranda Range. It was an uneventful drive until we arrived at the Barron River Bridge. I was explaining to Linda the agricultural District of Mareeba and failed to realize as I crossed the bridge that a gremlin was at work in the form of hand-waving, blue uniformed, policeman.

I look at my speedometer, only to see 72 kph as I drove past him. I was on the curvature of the road and felt that I needed a safe parking area on the grass verge, as traffic was rather heavy both ways. The officer then hopped into his car, did a u-turn and drove up behind me. I handed over my driving license and he walked back to his car to write out the traffic infringement (T.I.)

Waiting for his return I noticed that other vehicles had been pulled up at another police roadblock on the Kennedy Highway. The officer duly returned handed me the T.I. for $133 and two demerit points, with his congratulatory greetings of, "Happy Birthday for yesterday," Linda was suitably impressed.

I felt like Ricky Ponting stranded on 99. This was my first traffic infringement for speeding that blotted 49 years of driving and I just "Blew it and a year off 50!"

We arrived at the Scholls residence, had a great lunch amidst laughter and jokes that made up for the gremlin dilemma. We took our leave and drove back to see our Mareeba friends, Gloria and Ian Cowlard and their great dane, Carl, for afternoon tea.

Driving back home, the sun began to cast dark shadows through the rainforest trees of the Kuranda Range, it was a case of 'lights on' and drive carefully as the traffic had built up on the downhill journey.

Over the next couple of weeks we took Linda on several day trips and being adventurous she took herself to the Great Barrier Reef and to Green Island. She said, "I'm really delighted that I went, but when I reached Green Island I thought I was in little Japan, there were so many Japanese tourists on the Island." Linda had lived in Japan for some time after the World War II and had learnt to speak Japanese, "But I'm a little bit rusty now," she said.

Chapter 8
The Call

It's a Small World. Ring! Ring! I picked up the phone, announce myself, and listened to the person on the other end. I thank her and putting the phone down I turned to Nela and said, "We have to be down in Townsville Monday 27th for pre-admission into the hospital, as Tuesday the 28th April is 'D' Day and again I will be the first cab off the rank unless an emergency takes place." A letter dated 17th April confirmed the operation day. The long wait is over and finally it's on. Now we have to get moving and accomplish the things that need doing before our departure date from Cairns.

Leaving the women at home, I drive to the Cairns Base Hospital and made my way to the travel department located on the ground floor of 'B' Block. The receptionist gets my file from the filing cabinet and peruses the Travel Voucher that I had left with them previously.

The travel receptionist is very efficient and a few phone calls later I am advised that Nela and I are booked to travel on the Qantas (Sunstate) QF2305 Flight to Townsville on the 27th at 10:20am, and that a seat has been reserved for Linda who would travel with us. Linda said, "I'll be able to see some of Townsville tourist sights and to hold your hand when you need it." They also gave me a list of Motels to call for possible accommodation.

Having read through the provided list of things to take with me to the hospital I am glad that I had bought five sets of pj's, washed them and placed each set in individual, resealable plastic bags. I wanted to look my best when I walked around the hospital ward and it was easier for Nela to take them with her to wash and replace them in the bags. Little did I know that I would be wearing the hospitals very stylish, baggie grey pyjamas.

I jumped into my trusty steed the white Pajero before I headed for town and the Qantas booking office. Fortunately I find a vacant parking spot near the office, Oh no! No parking money! I rummage around and finally find 50 cents for the meter. I walk to the office, received a ticket for a customer service officer to call me then another short wait, pay for Linda's seat and collect our copy of the electronic ticket advice. How easy was that I thought?

The big question is where will Nela and Linda stay whilst I am in hospital? We have perused the list of possible motels, and whilst many state they are near the hospital we find that they are not within walking distance. They are not near a bus stop, and the only other way is by taxi and this would become very costly for a nine day stay or more. Even the motels were expensive and for pensioners, well I may need to sing on the street corner.

To our chagrin we discovered that Townsville was holding a sports carnival that weekend. Most of the motels were booked out. The motel area was in close proximity to the army barracks, the university and the hospital; and quite often the vacancies at that time were priceless! "What to do?" We mulled over the problem.

Meanwhile, Nela had to attend a meeting with her Filipina group. She mentioned our dilemma to Letty who had previously undergone an operation in Townsville over the Christmas period. "I stayed with a Filipino family for a few days after being discharged from hospital. Contact them and see if they can help," she said.

On arriving home that evening she contacted Mary-Ann Fein in Townsville and explained the situation about the accommodation. In the course of the conversation, Nela asked, "What part of the Philippines do you come from as I detect a Visayan accent?" Mary-Ann said, "I come from Hinigaran, Negros Occidental!"

Suddenly Nela erupted in the dialect and enthusiastically asked, "Where-in particular?" Well! Both are from the same hometown. They know or know of the people in the town and the telephone conversation took on a whole new meaning with much sighing and laughter. After an hour, Mary-Ann said, "Let me ask my husband something and I'll call you back shortly." The phone rang. "It's me again. I've asked my husband David, and you are most welcome to stay with us." "We have to get together and talk about our family background," Mary-Ann said. Nela was bubbling over with joy as she accepted their kind offer of accommodation. We could not thank her enough for their kind invitation. What a small world.

The next day Mary-Ann rang to say as she would be working upon our arrival in Townsville, she asked close friends, Randyll and Christine Armamento, another Filipino family to help us. Randyll would pick us up at the Airport because he would be babysitting their two boys Kurt and Neil as Christine, his wife, was a nurse on duty at the Hospital.

This brings out the best of the Filipinos, not only are they friendly and caring but they will go out of their way to accommodate you no matter how cramped for space. The children move into the family bedroom, sleep with each other or find a space on the floor to sleep and sacrifice their own comfort to make way for guests. They do so, without a murmur, as they are brought up to respect their elders, to be helpful and giving. They love life and do it with their continual smiles and laughter.

Chapter 9
The Flight

Time to Go. Listening to the announcement, "Would passengers flying from Cairns to Townsville on Qantas Flight 2305, please make your way to Gate 20 as your aircraft is now ready for boarding."

My mind begins to ponder and conjures up visual pictures of surgeons saying, 'Mr. Cortez, your bed is now ready for departure, climb aboard and be taken to Room 2 for the immediate withdrawal and renewal of your old aortic valve and while we are there we will replace your three, worn out arteries with new tubes.' But then! *Get that bugger Cortez down here now! So what, if he is in the loo! Rudd needs his bed.*

Perhaps, 'this is the last call for Mr. Cortez, we've looked everywhere in his chest but can't find him! Hold it! He's a one, slippery bugger; he was hiding behind the liver, get him and let's finish this op.'

I shake my head and readjust my mental picture of my surroundings in the airport departure lounge. We walk through the Gate and follow fellow passengers trudging along the safety fence and onto the tarmac to climb aboard the silver aluminum flying cigar!

It was a pleasant journey. A clear blue sky; occasionally we flew in and out of white, puffy clouds as we neared Townsville. Before we knew it the landing wheels are down and locked, and we glided down for a perfect landing onto the Townsville airstrip arriving at 11.15am. There was a slight breeze as we walked into the luggage pickup Area where we are met and greeted by Randyll and his two children Kurt and Neil. We again express our thanks for their kindness.

Time is on our side and we do not have to be at the hospital until 1:00pm. We ask Randyll to take us to the mall so that we can have a light lunch together. Randyll gives Nela his mobile number so that she can call him when she and Linda are ready to leave the hospital and go to Mary-Ann's house. After our lunch we clamber into his car and he drives us to the hospital.

Chapter 10
Townsville Hospital

It was one small step for Nela and Linda, one giant step for me as we walk through the portals of the Townsville Hospital. I am over-whelmed by the experience, especially since we had to wait previously for the telephone call all those long weeks ago.

In a flash, my mind navigates the brain cells producing electrical currents and I sift through all the informative overloads that I have read through to the coronary angiogram operation that has lead us here today. Yet! Here I am, feeling 100% fit and now facing an operation tomorrow morning. "What has destiny got in store for me?" I muse, as we continue our walk into the confines of the ground floor hospital building. I had expected just another hospital, but I was pleasantly surprised at this modern-day edifice. I wonder when Cairns will step up and build something similar, especially with the continual competitive hype between the two cities.

Then the question arises "but where?" We still need to maintain the present Cairns Base as a secondary hospital. Obviously the new hospital would be located south of Cairns, but by then, the population growth will have expanded immensely and the roadways which are bumper-to-bumper now will have expanded ten-fold to be a further headache for the motorist; no matter how many roads are built more cars will travel on them. It can be likened to the hospital bed problem no matter how many hospitals are built there will always be a bed problem.

The Townsville hospital has the space to expand; it incorporates the Townsville General Hospital and the Kirwan Hospital for Women. This is a first class hospital and it is also the largest hospital in provincial Australia that supports the local Community as well as people in the North to Thursday Island and Papua New Guinea, West to Mount Isa and South to Sarina.

I have learnt that, 'it is also a major teaching hospital of the James Cook University School of Medicine and is closely affiliated with the

University of Queensland and James Cook University.'

'The Townsville Hospital provides a comprehensive healthcare environment that has been designed with a patient-friendly approach to layout and location of services. The clustering of services from the same disciplines as well as the new model of care promotes familiarity with staff and easy access for patients and their families.' (www.health.qld.gov.au/townsville/Facilities/tville_hosp.asp)

Well the die is cast! I now have a general feeling of the hospital, and wait for the medical staff to wave their magic wand over all the patients for a successful outcome. I don't need to get stressed out and worry myself sick. I'll leave it for the experts who are each following their own destinies in the field of medicine.

Chapter 11
Pre-Admission

The Little Steps. Having taken that giant step, I cautiously take the small steps as I walk towards the Central Admissions Reception Desk. The admission time is set for 1.00pm but being a stickler for time we are 15 minutes early.

The receptionist smiles, takes my name and particulars and then tells me to take a seat until my name is called. Some 20 minutes later, I hear my name, looking up I notice a woman standing outside her door, she directs us into her office that is no bigger than a shoe-box, but it serves its purpose with a desk, chairs and computer.

The admin officer asks me quite a number of questions, gives me some forms which I duly sign and hands me further information papers that includes a step-by-step guide to your hospital visit – cardiac surgery and information booklet.

She informs me that the guide, "will help you understand what you can expect during your stay in hospital for your recovery from surgery. However, it is intended as a guide and may vary for each individual."

We are told to make our way to the elevator and to follow the directions that were given to us. Of course, we got lost, but we follow the crumbs like Hansel and Gretel and finally reach our destination. Approaching the Med 3 Reception desk I am met with friendly smiles from several nurses as I introduce myself, Nela and Linda. We are asked to take a seat as my bed is not yet available; we welcome this and take the time to peruse the booklets that we had recently received.

Chapter 12
Pre-Surgery Tests

Overload. Walking into the sterile environment of the Med 3 Ward my mind is alive with shooting stars that create meteors of thoughts of what I can expect in the hours and days ahead of me.

I am shown to my corner bed with a large window that overlooks the green shrubbery outside and the hospital filled car park where people are casually or hurrying along the pathways.

Nela and Linda are suitably impressed with the outlook and the ultra-cleanliness of the ward. They sit in the comfortable chairs beside the bed and quietly talk whilst I divest my bag of my clothing and toiletry items that are placed in the bedside cabinet. Having finished unpacking, I sit on the bed and we discuss what is about to happen for the rest of the afternoon.

We are interrupted by a nurse who asks my name; where I am and what type of surgery I will under-go. I discovered in the days ahead that I will answer these questions on numerous occasions, this is understandable. I can see the security and the safety of ensuring that the right person has the right operation, at the right time. This is okay by me as I really don't want a hair transplant, when I should have had a new valve! Having perused the Cardiac Surgery Guide booklet, I am visibly impressed with the wide variety of people who will be involved with me before and after my surgery.

Oh, my! The vampire has arrived and while she will not give me that fatal neck kiss, so often shown at the movies, she will stick a needle into me and draw blood. I tend to look away showing little interest, but flinched internally as the needle penetrates the vein in my left arm, I cannot help myself and look at the blood being withdrawn into the hypodermic syringe.

Another nurse subjects me to a blood pressure test, then proceeds to take my temperature, pulse, respiration rate, my height and weight all of which is recorded on my medical sheet.

To make sure that I do not get lost or kidnapped by some of the attractive nurses roaming the hospital corridors, a second nurse places a plastic identification bracelet with my name on it around my right wrist. The surgeons do not really want to operate on another person apart from me during their quest of opening me up and checking for unaccountable, hidden bodies.

Enter the young, female physiotherapist who makes her appearance without any fanfare and begins to tell me her role towards my recovery stage.

Apparently, as soon as I awake from my forced slumber I will be subjected to breathing exercises via the use of the Voldyne/triflow, it is a three-sectional, plastic valve like-apparatus that may have come from outer space. The aim of the game being to inhale and maintain the float between the designated blue markings, fortunately it is not a breathalyzer. I will need to do this exercise at least six times every hour, no worries I can do it! Famous last words, try it after the operation I exhaled rather than inhaled and of course, got nowhere. However, as each day passes the exercise becomes easier.

"How do you like dressing up?" She asks with a smile on her face. I asked, "Why?" "Because you will need to wear these white stockings on both legs, this is to improve circulation and to prevent or reduce the risk of blood clots forming in the veins of the legs." I could just visualize myself wearing the white stockings with shorts and a white shirt, shades of my life in Papua New Guinea. How chic, but, what the heck.

The next exercise was getting up from the bed or chair with my arms crossed over my chest and using a one, two rocking motion and up on three! Fortunately I had read about this exercise after I saw Dr Tam in Cairns and I began doing the exercises on a regular basis until it became an automatic response. Try doing it when you're on the loo, a funny experience.

There will be no room for, 'let me lie here.' You will need to get up and start your short walks around the nurse's station; this will be the order of the day. The physio has set the goals and it is up to me to do the breathing and walking exercises in order to gain a full recovery after the operation.

The pharmacist explains her role and will provide the medication as per the doctor's instruction. In the meantime I have handed over my medication to the nurse who records them on my chart. She tells me, "They will be under lock and key and will be administered at the appropriate time with any new medication."

Ironically, before seeing Dr Tam, Nela had borrowed a book from the Cairns Library entitled "Death by Prescription". It mentions that many people jump from doctor to doctor and each in their own mind prescribe medication as per the symptoms of the patient. The patient cannot remember the name of the medication but describes the colors to the doctor. The author advocated making a list on the computer with the patient and the doctor's name, address, telephone number and the name and dosage of the present medication. When asked what type of medication they take, it is a matter of taking the list out of your wallet and handing it to the doctor. Both Nela and I have ours in our wallets and it really helps to have the information at hand.

Food! Wonderful food! I salivate at the thought of my favourite food but I'm gently brought back to earth when the dietician tells me that I will be on a low fat diet, given water and fluids, and a meal within a day or so after having my surgery. Do you believe this! Then she tells me that, "there might be a loss of appetite for a short while and that the taste of food will be different." I'm already looking forward to a home-cooked meal. Oh, well! It's nice to be told that I will be on a diet and it is something I had not expected.

The Education Rehabilitation Coordinator makes a brief stop-over and provides information for my recovery and will advise when I would join a group to watch a video that outlines ways and the various needs for a healthy life after the surgery.

Wake up! Wake up! I'll probably hear the dulcet voices of angels urging me to open my eyes, but the Anaesthetist has made an appearance to tell me that since I'm having an aortic valve replacement and a triple by-pass, a general anaesthetic would be used. This is a mixture of drugs that will keep me unconscious and pain-free during the operation. He further explains that during the surgery different drugs will be given at particular times for a specific purpose. I can well imagine waking up and yelling "yeehah!"

I tell him that I have a dental bridge and that I have been having a nasal discharge that leaves a sticky substance in my mouth and throat. He makes note of the information then looks at my list of medication and notes that I am taking aspirin; that I don't smoke nor drink and that I had worked to increase my fitness when I realized that I would need an operation. He further tells me that modern anaesthesia is very safe. However, risks do occur. If things are meant to happen, they will happen and since I have no control over anything then I am not going to stress out!

Time is ticking away and Nela, Linda and I are breathless with all the overload that we have experienced in a short time but it hasn't ended, a nurse arrives with an orderly who is pushing a wheelchair. I ask, "Where am I going?" In reply, she said, "You need a chest x-ray taken and an ECG that traces your heart rhythm also needs to be done." I said, "I'm okay and I can walk there!" "Sorry the wheel chair is for you," she replied. The ECG and the chest x-ray are taken and I am wheeled back to the ward. Fortunately, there are no traffic accidents as we negotiate our return trip along well lit corridors.

The ward nurse informs me that at 6.00am next morning I will be woken up and that I will have a body shave (by a male nurse). I will then shower twice using the special antibacterial solution to wash my whole body prior to going into surgery.

She then tells me that all my clothing should be packed into my bag as these will be placed in a secured office, my toiletries, stockings and the voldyne breathing machine will be taken to the surgical intensive care area. So after carefully putting things into the bedside cabinet I now have to take them out again and repack them into my bag. She further mentions that I would not be returning to this ward but will be going across the corridor. Oh, well! I had a pleasant view for a short time! I'm further advised that the doctors will be around to see me in the early evening.

It is now approaching 5.30pm and I tell Nela to ring Randyll for him to pick her up outside the hospital so that he can drive both of them to Mary-Ann's house. Before leaving she asks the nurse what time would be the best to come into the hospital before I'm taken to the operating theatre; they are told to be at Med 3 before 7.00am. Randyll calls to say that he is downstairs waiting for them; hugs and kisses and they take their leave.

It's been a really long afternoon and the meteors that had been whizzing around my mind have gone into information overload. However, it is not over yet as the team doctors assisting Dr Tam are due to see me after the evening meal.

They arrive about 7.30pm and entering my bed space they pulled the white curtains closed for some privacy. They introduce themselves as Drs Rajiv and Alveska. The inevitable questions arise – what is your name? etc. "They ask me what kind of operation I am going to have and the type of valve I had decided on." I mentioned that I had told Dr Tam I would go for the mechanical valve but I still had reservations about the "warfarin" medication that had to be taken for life and the constant

41

monitoring of the required levels.

The female doctor explained in depth the effects of the warfarin and the types of valves that are used. The explanation provided me with more information that enabled me to reassess my previous decision. This new information pushed me to alter my decision; I changed my mind and decided to go with the Mitral Valve Tissue replacement. I had no qualms about my new decision. Did it worry me? No! The Doctors were surprised and they asked, "Are you sure?" In reply I answered, "Yes."

Decisions! Decisions! Life is full of them some easy and others more difficult; but we make them and often than not we are winners.

We are all humans and life is short, but medical technology and procedures are changing in leaps and bounds, and by the time I reach a life expectancy of 85 years the world would have under-gone a myriad of changes in the medical field. Hopefully, I may forestall a major operation in my twilight years!

They reassured me that I would come out a new man and an increase in life expectancy; however, there was a very small percentage that things could go wrong. I said, "I have no control over the operation, you are the experts. I'm an avid fan of the TV show RPA (Royal Prince Alfred) and know that you will give of your best. Just make sure that you cut straight!" Both doctors again questioned me about my decision to change and I told them I was happy with the tissue valve replacement. They wished me a pleasant sleep and left me digesting what we had discussed.

The one thing the day's events showed me is that, it is not the name of the individual person, but the importance of a group of dedicated medical staff that work towards a common goal of a "team" effort, in caring and helping the patient overcomes their inner stress before surgery.

On pondering what I had witnessed and gained, I realize that I'm just one patient out of many who have under-gone or will under-go similar surgery. Imagine if you would, and multiply the number of patients in a day, a week, a month, a year or more and you will understand the amount of work the dedicated medical staff do to improve our way of life. What would we do without them?

Time is marching on and the ward nurse tells me that I will be wakened up at 6.00am for a full body shave and at 7.00am I will travel the corridors to the operating theatre. I change into my pj's and go through half-an-hour of deep breathing exercises beside the window; this allows me to clear my mind and ensures that I have a goodnight's sleep.

Don't stress out if you are not in control of things.

Chapter 13
The Countdown

Bling! Bling! I am aroused by my internal alarm. I open my eyes and gaze around at the soft, light beams that are filtering through the gaps of the window curtain. Glancing at my watch I note that it has just turned 5.30 am and a thought jumps into my mind, *this is the day. This is the countdown. This will be a heart stopper.*

I slowly eased out of my bed coverings and slipped out of bed then headed for the bathroom where I washed my face, brushed my teeth and combed my hair. I'll shower after I receive my full body shave I thought upon returning to my bed.

Since I am the only patient in the Ward I do not hesitate and open the curtains to let a new day of sunshine stream into the room but it is still dark and the light that I saw was from the outside path lights. Standing and looking outside, I closed my eyes and begin my deep breathing and extending Ki (energy) exercises; within a short time I begin to sense the rising of the dawn as darkness gives way to light without a care in the world.

Twenty minutes into the exercise I am brought back to normality by a gentle cough behind me and a voice apologizing for the interruption. 'It is the Barber of Seville.' I think as I wind down my exercises. He tells me his name, and I apologize for it is a name now long forgotten and says, "I'm your barber for today," as he throws a sheet over the bed to ensure that he catches all the hair clippings. Then he closes the curtains surrounding my bed. He asks me to strip and to lay face down, and then drapes a towel over my rear end.

The hum of the clipper is like a miniature lawnmower as it does its job in removing the hair from my back, then it is time to turn over as the clipper continues its journey through the grasslands of my body. It is a 72 year old specimen of a body that showed a semblance of compact muscles of yesteryear. The pecs show some muscle but the stomach bumps of, 'stout Cortez,' belies the former structure of a once lean, sleek

Adonis (I wish!)

I am in a relaxed state but occasionally wince as the cutter snags and tugs on some unruly, wiry chest hair. A few more swipes and the ordeal is over. The male orderly brushes away the loose hair and tells me that I can now go for my shower.

Taking the sexy hospital gown, I head for the bathroom and following the instructions of how to use the antibacterial solution I take two showers to make sure that all the loose hair is washed down the drain and that I have a clean body. Having already shaved and brushed my teeth again, I unfurl the gown like a Spanish matador of old, and slip into its slinky folds looking like all other patients who have donned the same hospital specialty as a member of the hospital choir singing, *this is the moment, the moment I trust,* for it is the countdown for the surgeons I trust, as I leave the bathroom.

In the meantime, Nela and Linda have arrived from Mary-Ann's house. I tell them about the discussions I had with the two Doctors the night before. Nela is rather peeved that she had missed the meeting and was concerned over my last minute decision to change from the mechanical valve to the Mitroflow Tissue Heart Valve. I mention that the change was further based on information and in particular the warfarin medication. I told her not to worry as I was happy and only the future will tell if my decision for change was correct.

The ward nurse arrives to give me a short medication tablet that helps me to relax and makes me drowsy, and within time sends me off to "la la" land. I am told to stay on my bed and just after 7.00am I am taken on a grand tour of the hospital corridors with overhead lighting flashing by and with Nela and Linda in tow behind me I am wheeled to the theatre.

Before entering the portals of the theatre I meet the theatre nurse who asks the inevitable questions, 'What is your name? What kind of operation will you have? What is the date of your birthday?' Groggily I answer the questions but it's like a game of monopoly; *You have just received your 'Get out of Goal' free card, or move three steps back as there is another emergency more important than yours, or congratulations move forward two steps and you will have your operation,* I muse over in my drowsy state.

I'm given the expected hugs, kisses and words of endearment, "I love you!" "I love you too!" Then the doors open and close behind me as I am wheeled into a clinical environment and a new countdown begins before the operation commences.

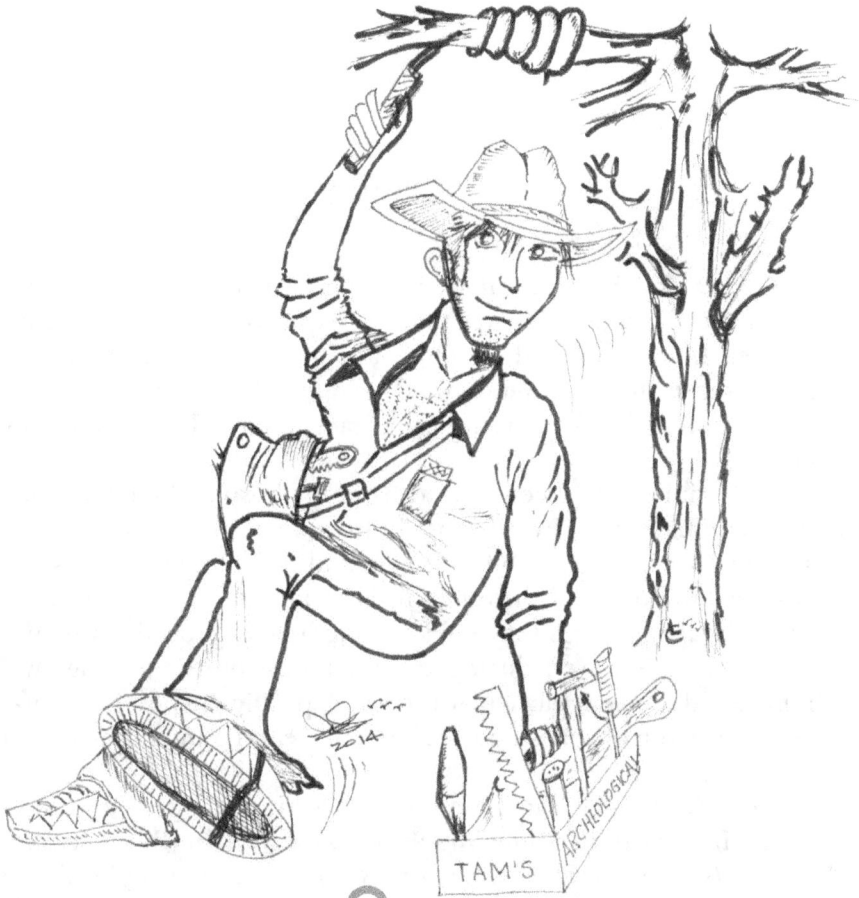

Chapter 14
The Knockout

Oink! Oink! There is a quiet air of expectancy in the operating theatre that is filled with a high level of medical expertise, such as the surgeons, anaesthetist, nurses and the technicians to run the bypass machine. I groggily sense the confidence that pervades the inner strength of all who are about to perform a surgical miracle on me. Thank God they are experts.

By the time I had been moved from my hospital bed and onto the operating table I had already lapsed into a deep sleep. The anaesthetist has done an admirable job in attaching all his plumbing lines for the anaesthetic to flow freely through my body and to refresh your memory; 'It is a mixture of drugs that will keep me in a state of unconsciousness and pain-free, however, during the operation different drugs will be administered to me at particular times for specific purposes.' Thankfully we do not run out of anaesthetic! (National Heart Foundation of Australia Booklet p6)

Sleep! Sleep! The knockout punch has hit me and I am in the land of nod. Harking back to my initial interview with Dr Tam I had asked, "Will I be on the operating table for six hours considering I will have an aortic valve replacement and a triple bypass? He smiled and said, "No, it will take about three hours and we will have two teams working side by side each other."

I can only surmise that my intrepid adventurers are likened to a group of archaeologists within the realms of the medical solar system who will delve into the nooks and crannies, deep within the sinkhole of my opened chest. I sense that the hands will slip and slide amidst a pool of red claret a gentle, gurgling sound emanates from the hand-held vacuum that sucks the areas clean. Allowing them to investigate, detect and diagnose the locality of repair or even discover an unwanted alien lurking in an unexpected area.

Team 2 under the direction of Drs Rajiv and Aleska have abseiled down perilous slopes onto the newly shorn left leg, where they have plotted and marked the least line of resistance before they make their incision to find the elusive, slippery vein, that lies beneath the inner area of the knee to the mid-point of the ankle.

The team's mission is to, 'Perform one or more cuts on the leg and remove the vein for the by-pass graft canals. Sometimes the cut is also made from the groin so that the larger blood vessels can be reached.' (National Heart Foundation of Australia Booklet 6). If it hurts I won't feel a thing!

Team 2 has successfully found the clear, thin slippery vein and tying off each end of the required length they make their cut. Placed in a bowl of anti-bacterial solution it is washed and cleaned. The 'A' Team now has a vein worthy of replacing the three blocked arteries within me. In fact, most mothers would be proud of their prowess, as they plied the needle with a flourish in sewing an invisible line as they re-attach the skin flaps of the leg together.

Meanwhile the 'A' Team under the guidance and the mentoring of Dr Tam watch in awe as he 'ensures his cut is true through the midline of the chest through the breastbone (sternum) to reach the heart. During surgery my body is kept cool to protect the vital organs by slowing down their working rate so that they need less oxygen. A heart-lung machine takes over the function of the heart and lungs. (National Heart Foundation of Australia Booklet p6).

I slumber on as Dr Tam and his team work methodically and without haste, towards a successful outcome in replacing the aortic valve and the triple by-pass grafts. I was reassured in previous discussion before the operation that, 'If I needed a blood transfusion, all blood products used for the transfusion in Australia are strictly screened to protect patients against viruses that can cause hepatitis and Aids. (National Heart Foundation of Australia Booklet p7). What a relief to know that stringent security checks are in place for all blood products!

After three or more hours, both teams have performed their usual surgical miracle and now they have wired my sternum together again, using titanium wire and within six months the bone structure will have calcified over the wire making the breastbone even stronger. They have plied the needle once in sewing my chest together with precision. They are flaming geniuses.

Technology in the medical world today, has come forward in leaps and bounds, but belies the surgeon's skill in manipulating such a slippery, thin, bugger of a vein that defies the lay man's comprehension in using microscopic surgery, but they do and I congratulate them all!

Through their efforts I have now become a member of the illustrious club, "The Oink! Oink! Tissue Valve Fraternity," Hurrah! For those who have gone before me, you now belong to an elite group of people who have received extra years to their lives through medical surgery and technology. You are in a league of your own and can now belong to one of three fraternities; the Oink! Oink! (Pig) Moo! Moo! (Bovine) or the Clunk! Clunk! (Mechanical) Take ownership now.

Barring possible problems, when I awake from my deep slumber *I will have a new lease on life that will see me through my post-op recovery.* Intensive Care Unit here I come!

Chapter 15
The Intensive Care Unit

Wake up! Wake up! I'm oblivious to my surroundings within the walls of the intensive care unit (ICU) and continue to slumber on, without a care in the world.

Meanwhile it is 3.00pm in the afternoon of Tuesday 28th April and Nela has called to see what time was convenient for Linda and her to visit me. The ward receptionist replies, "You can come over now."

In a blink of an eye she and Linda have hopped onto their magic carpet and soaring through the afternoon skies land within the realms of the ICU only to be confronted with an image of a futuristic alien from outer space.

They gaze upon a body that was energetic, vibrant and a picture of health only 24 hours ago. To one that now has a multitude of plastic tubes protruding from the torso. In the space of seconds, they take in the breathing tube hanging from my mouth that helps me to breathe while still asleep from the anaesthetic. At the other end of the spectrum they see a catheter tube that is covered by a sheet that leads into a bottle; this line fulfils the need of my bladder. They see lines jutting from the neck area and are told that these are the central venous line and catheter that is used for the infusion of drugs and fluids, and for monitoring venous pressures. My left arm lies on the crisp, white sheet and from the wrist, the arterial line hangs limply but it monitors my blood pressure and for taking blood samples; drain tubes and the pacing wire emerges from my lower chest. Stuck to this robotic chest they see the six, white electrodes that are attached to a monitor that provides further information as to my well-being! Beep! Beep!

They take note of the unfamiliar sounds that emanate from the monitors and the ventilator alarm that stand majestically around the bed, with blood pressure cuffs and a box of surgical gloves. But I am still in a deep sleep and not concerned with the probable bustle of human behavior in my new environmental surroundings.

However, the dulcet voice of the ward angel extols me to wake up. "Loury wake up! Nela is here! Your cousin Linda is here! Wake up! All for naught!" Nela asks, "Is there something wrong?" In reply, the nurse said, "No everything is ok, we just need him to breathe for himself and not the machine. You can tell from the monitor if Loury is breathing alright it will indicate high and if he isn't, the machine the level will be low."

Nela chimes in with her wake up call, followed by the American twang from Linda, "Loury wake up! Wake up! Look at this beautiful, blonde nurse who is calling you," but to no avail I am deep in slumber land. Their chorus continues for some time and they jump for joy each time I reach a high level, then their smiles drop as once again the breathing level falls. Unfortunately, dusk arrives and they must leave me for the night until they return next morning to see if this spaced out alien has returned to mother earth. Another chapter waits.

Chapter 16
Day 1 Post Op

Open Eyes. A spell has been cast and the alien continues to sleep, but it is time to awaken the human within, open eyes, to see the reflective lights above and the shadows bouncing off the walls and the human activity within the intensive care unit.

Nela and Linda arrived mid-morning and together with the nurse, the three divas begin their awakening chorus of wake up, "Loury! Wake up! Open your eyes!"

My senses are dimmed, but, a voice deep inside me, tells me to wake up; unfortunately my eyes are glued shut and I am unable to open them. However, their serenading continues and something is breaking through my unconsciousness and I will myself to move my fingers, to nod my head. The girls notice my movement of acknowledgement and are elated as they continue to speak those famous words of wake up, open your eyes.

I slowly awake from the darkness and begin to see the light, as my eyelids become unglued and quiver to make out blurred images around me, that sluggishly take the shape of human figures. I try to turn my head and to take in these ghostly figures, but the breathing tube prevents me from achieving that simple goal.

My memory of the operation is zilch! I reopen my tired eyes, but I am not able to speak nor can I eat or drink because of the breathing tube in my mouth. I am still receiving an infusion of pain-relieving drugs, but apart from the drowsiness I am not feeling any pain. I am assured by the nurse that if I have any pain, it will decrease when the chest drains are removed within 24 to 48 hours. Nodding my head drowsily in acknowledgement I try to smile but instead see the smiles and relief on the faces of Nela and Linda. They tell me much later that they were concerned but were happy that I had a successful operation.

The ICU doors spring open and a bed is trundled across the floor towards me, the nurse informs me that I will be moved onto it and taken to Med 3. A host of activities begin to surround me, the nurses have noted that I am breathing quite strong and the doctor has given his approval to remove the breathing tube from my mouth. Relief! Although I am still in a stupor I am now able to talk or is it mutters, through a cotton-filled mouth to those around me. The plumbing and drainage tubes are lifted to ensure that they do not snag during my short flight onto the Med 3 bed.

Nela has decided to help, and makes a move towards removing a drink bottle from atop of the bedside cabinet. Apparently and in a gruff voice, I said, "Don't do that!" She was quite peeved that having gone through an operation and still dazed with sleep, that I could tell her off! I don't remember a thing but it must have been the alien residing in my body. I apologize for hurting her feelings at that time and blame it on a sudden mood swing. My mind was still in a stupor so what was I thinking? What made me say it? No idea!

It is near midday when I once again follow the ceilings and walls whilst being propelled along corridors and corners to reach my final destination of Med 3 where I will languish for the next seven to nine days. Nevertheless to be rejuvenated with exercise and the charisma of the nurses who will help towards my recovery?

I am wheeled into a ward and expect to see the puzzled looks of the male patients who think to themselves, 'Here's another one!' Alas, I am confronted by members of the fairer sex, who think, 'What is this guy doing here amongst us women, and how long will we have to put up with him?' However, in reality they smile at me, some say hi and then go back to musing over their own thoughts for the day.

They must have sighed with relief when several hours later I am moved into the next ward and look upon my male counterparts, another alien has arrived! Luck is with me as the bed now occupies a corner with a full size window that lets light into the ward and allows me to look out onto a small, tree-lined path complete with other humans walking to and fro.

Nela and Linda have gone for the day to enable me to rest up, ha! I believe a bevy of medical personnel will be coming my way shortly to follow-up what I need to do in pushing my recovery along.

My recovery regimen begins with the physiotherapist who has arrived to take me through the 'voldyne' breathing machine exercises. She tells me that I need to reach the 1000 level and it needs to be done every hour. I feel like the wolf and the three pig's tale of old, huff and puff! Quite an experience when you are still drowsy! She tells me that tomorrow I will be taking small steps and by the end of the program I am expected to climb a set of stairs. I am reminded not to put pressure through my arms when getting in and out of bed. If I cough or sneeze, my huggie pillow is my first line of defense that needs to be held it tightly against my chest to help stop the movement against the pain that beats within the surgical site. Fortunately I was only faced with small dry coughs.

I look a treat with my hospital pj's and adorning my legs, the brilliant, white TED stockings, that helps to improve circulation and minimizes the fluid accumulation in the legs. Rest assured this will provide me the basis for an effective and early exercise program. Oh! For my sun-tanned legs again.

The ward nurse makes her way to my bed carrying a weighing machine. It is time to weigh myself, so with the remote control I lower the bed to its lowest point. She helps me to swing my legs over the edge and clutching my huggie pillow I do the 1, 2 and up movement to stand; what an ordeal for the first time! Standing on the machine I am a little unsteady on my feet but I accomplish the feat with her help and from 83 kgs I have lost some weight.

It is also time to measure my blood pressure and pulse rate, and after the cuff is placed around my upper arm I can watch and read the results on the monitor, however with drooping eyelids I show little interest but accept that all is well. This test will continue every one to two hours, I am told.

The Dr Rajiv has paid me a visit, to see how I am faring and will continue to see me with his entourage each day to check on my progress

I sip from my bottled water, but need to take more than a sip. I am a firm believer of drinking eight glasses of water per day because it has certainly helped me ward off the dreaded gout, I believe! One of my recovery goals is to ensure that I drink a lot of water. The other is to become physically fit by walking and doing light leg exercises. To the latter I visualize myself being a soldier in training! Left! Right! Left!

I have put the bed on an incline to help me sit upright and to be able to reach the bottle of water; reading is out of the question as I am unable to concentrate; so it is a matter of looking around at the other patients, gazing out of the window or closing my eyes.

Fortunately or unfortunately, there are breaks in these little activities, especially when it is time for my tablets as I need to take them every four hours, or as the Doctor prescribed on my chart. I have asked the nurse to forgo the painkiller medication as I am not suffering any pain. She agrees and notes it on my chart with the proviso that they will reappear if any pain suddenly erupts within my body! In the meantime, having a new aortic valve, I now need to take a warfarin tablet that will treat and prevent blood clots. 'How many more pills will I need to captivate with my smile before I leave the medical portals of the Hospital?' I ask myself. A tablet here, a tablet there! And by the time I am discharged I will be sick and tired of them.

Eating is out of the question at the moment as I do not have the appetite for it, but I realize that it is the only way to build up my energy. However, sleep comes around early! I now have to attempt to sleep the whole night through on my back! What will the morning bring as I pull the blanket up to my neck?

Chapter 17
Day 2 Post Op

Shuffle Steps. The lights are switched on, curtains are drawn and there is an air of activity in the ward. I am able to open my eyes slowly, despite the eyelids being heavy with sleep. It is not because of the anaesthetic, but being woken in the early hours of the morning to partake in a feast of medication tablets! However, it is an extra tablet once more! I am given a potassium supplement and a lasix tablet that slows a fluid buildup; these are but two of the other eight that I force down with copious gulps from the water bottle.

I look around and watch my new found friends stirring from their broken sleep, all wishing that they could slumber on a few more hours. I see with interest the grimace on each face, as they subject themselves to the same ordeal of swallowing their issue of the brightly, coloured tablets that make the journey down the throat canal to the stomach. What a perilous ride they take.

The breakfast trolley arrives, and each of us received our tray of food. Since I did not put in my order, I face the prospect of downing a bowl of porridge. I clumsily take the lid off the orange juice container and sip the contents without taste. Next the packet of milk is opened and I nearly drop it due to my awkward handling, but I gain control and I saturate the now semi-cold porridge. I tend to play around with it as it is not my first choice of cereal. Nevertheless there is a need to sustain myself believing it is delicious by putting spoon to mouth, fighting through its blandness and its presentation, ugh! Fortunately, I am in heaven, as I gaze upon my favourite fruit, the banana.

I tackle the very cold dinner roll by cutting it into two, and then I lather it with a small packet of butter and a packet of strawberry jam. Yeah, I know, I've just had an operation and a deadly cholesterol agent may infest my organs, but how sweet it is! I wash this down with a mug of tepid tea that I produced from a tea bag that accompanies the breakfast tray.

Breakfast is over and I stare vacantly out the window for a short time. However, I am brought back to earth when the nurse arrives with two towels and a set of fresh pj's. "It is time to have your shower, but we need to disconnect your plumbing lines first," she said.

My urinary catheter is removed. My ECG monitor is disconnected and the pacing wire that rests on my heart is left in, but it is covered and taped down onto my chest. The drip and drains disappear and the futuristic alien of 24 hours ago has been transformed into a human form once again. To enable the nurse to dispose of the dressing that has covered my leg wound the TED stockings have been removed under duress. She said, "After you have your shower, we will let the wound dry off before putting on a new sterile dressing." For the first time I am able to see the snake-like incision where the vein was removed and the cut has been resewn. I wonder how long before the scar disappears, nevertheless I am no longer an alien and perhaps it will not disappear completely or will it?

Although the bed is at a 45 degree angle, I find it difficult to move my leaden legs to the side and I require help from the nurse. She has lowered the bed to its lowest point making it easier for me to stand-up. Finally my legs dangle from the bed where I can do my balancing act whilst the nurse stands ready to catch me should I overbalance and free-fall to the floor. Since I need to hug my small pillow and unable to put pressure on my arms to push up from the bed, it is a case of the 1, 2 and up movement once more and this rocking to and fro will continue for many weeks into my recovery at the hospital and eventually when I return home.

I meander across the room like a drunken sailor to the bathroom and with her help my short, shuffling steps take me to my destination. Upon entering the inner sanctum of this holy washroom her dulcet voice tells me what to do. More importantly the necessity and the use of the anti-bacterial body cleanser solution. It is the first time in my life that I needed to sit down to have a shower as my legs were still unsteady. The hot water is heavenly, but all good things come to an end! Then the question arises as the water trickles down my body to the drain below, 'How do I dry myself?'

I haven't the strength or the agility to dry myself down. I look around and spy the help button; pushing it I find myself in heaven and framed in the doorway three angels appear. They have come to my rescue. I ask them hoarsely, "Where were you when I was 21 years old?" Giggling they replied, "We weren't even born then!" Oh, the agony!

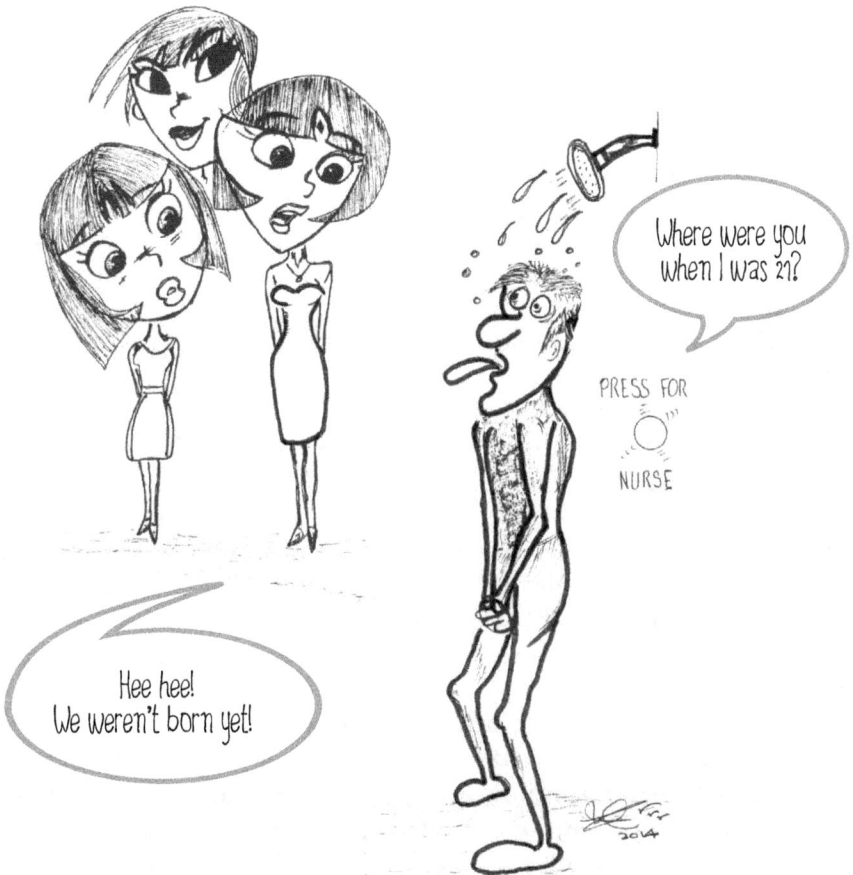

Dressed in clean pj's, I soft shoe-shuffle back from the bathroom to my bed and sit down. Yet again I need the nurse's assistance in moving my legs onto the bed. The activity has sapped my energy, I ask the nurse to settle the pillows behind my back and as I struggle to get comfortable my eyelids become heavy. Unfortunately, sleep evades me and I watch a nurse pushing a trolley towards me that is laden with vials. I see a picture of a vampire and realize the blood-sucking nurse has arrived to give me that delightful love kiss! I could be so lucky! No way! Grinning she says, "I'm back."

With a gleam in her eyes she tightens the strap around my bicep then tells me to make a fist. Tapping my arm just above the elbow she looked for that elusive vein; finding it she swabs the area, saying, "This will be a little prick, oops I mean sting!" Political correctness rears its ugly head once more! We can say, the 's' word or the 'f' word but using the 'p' word is out of the question. I am mystified! I thank her as she covers the puncture in my arm. She tells me that the test will check my potassium level and the clotting ability of my blood. 'What did they do in the old days?' I mused.

Sometime later, the ward nurse gives me another pin prick, oops, in my abdomen. The injection will help 'thin' my blood, but I believe I have taken warfarin which does the same thing or was it later? So, let's hope it doesn't over-thin the blood that is coursing through my body and seep out through all the ongoing pinpricks.

The cuff is wrapped around my upper arm, the monitor button is pressed and the magic of technology computes my blood pressure and pulse "All is well," said the smiling nurse as she records the figures onto my chart together with my oxygen saturation level reading that also proves to be okay.

Half-an-hour later she returns with a bottle of betadine antiseptic solution that she swabs over my leg wound followed by a fresh sterile dressing. With great gusto she stretches and huffs and puffs in pulling on the ever-so tight TED stockings onto both legs. 'What an effort' I thought! Will Nela be able to do the same especially with her weak wrists, but time will tell?'

Having reached one goal I am confronted with another. I struggle once more off the bed to have myself weighed, only to discover a further weight loss. Since I am now in an upright position I decided to go for my shuffling, constitutional walk but not far! It is rather amusing to see grown men making their journey along the corridor, carrying their most trusted, important huggie pillow. Without it, a sudden cough or sneeze and the pain will be excruciating. Fortunately, I do not have the inclination to cough or sneeze nor am I suffering any pain.

Every hour on the hour I inhale through my extraterrestrial, breathing apparatus and try to reach the 1500 level that has been set for me, but my breathing is jerky and I am unable to hold the level! It will come with perseverance and as my deep breathing improves. To help the breathing I try a few light coughs to clear my chest whilst hugging my wonderful pillow; it hurts a little, with no serious pain, yet I will survive. Life was never so good!

One of my new found friends has left leaving a vacant bed space, but miraculously another bed reappears! What magic this hospital holds.

My light lunch has come and gone and I expect to see Nela and Linda around 3.00pm after my short rest period. The recliner chair beside my bed beckoned me, although I try to move to it I must again seek help from the nurse! What a wimp! Limbs must be functional to move, whereas mine were in a leaden state. I finally reached my desired object as pillows are placed behind and a blanket thrown over me, but I ask once more for the nurse to raise the footrest. I thank her profusely and give her my best smile. Feeling comfortable I doze off, only to be wakened for another bout of pill swallowing, ugh! A necessary evil for all who have travelled the same path of recovery!

Nela has tracked down the small kitchenette and armed with their piping hot coffee they arrive at my bedside. They settle down and tell me that they had gone to watch the IMAX movie, had their light lunch and visited the Townsville Aquarium. They said, "We've had a great day that was interesting and informative." They are enjoying their stay with Mary-Anne and the family, and consider themselves lucky that the Bus Stop is right outside their front door.

I tell them of my adventures of the past several hours and that I was waiting for the young, female physiotherapist who will assess my breathing exercises and walking skills of an unsteady, shuffling 72 year old man; both laughed.

It is surprising, how talking saps away one's energy but our conversations continue as we rattle on. A phone call tells them that Randyll is waiting downstairs to drive them back to Mary-Ann's house. So with hugs and kisses they make their way to the car park. Our new found friends are a god-send! What would we do without them?

Cousin Linda is due to fly back to Cairns on Friday and will be picked-up by my son Darren and Dannille from the airport. She will spend two days at home then fly via Sydney to New Zealand to meet with one of her best friends, and after a relaxing and cold week, she will be homeward bound for Seattle, USA.

The physio arrives and checks my breathing and takes me for a short walk where I meet other familiar faces with each of us carrying our huggie pillows. She tells me that I am doing well but not to over-do it. "Remember you have just had an operation." With those motivational words transmitted along my brain waves, she leaves and I sink back into the recliner.

Much later I need to go to the bathroom, but I do not have the strength to push down the foot rest and once again call upon the nurse for her help. She arrives and kneels down on the floor to push it in. This caused me some embarrassment because of the strain she used on her shoulders and back, especially when you consider work, health and safety policies. I vowed that I would work out a better way of becoming more independent, rather than rely on the nurses that have more important things to do. Yes, I understand that they have a job to do but I am safety conscious and I would rather not have a nurse pull a muscle so that I can be more comfortable!

The arrival of Dr Rajiv and his retinue of observers, signaled the pulling of the curtains around my bed to ensure some privacy during my interview. He asked whether I was suffering any pain or soreness. I answered in the negative but told him that I had some numbness in my left wrist where a cannula had been inserted, and also around my left leg where the vein had been taken. "In time the numbness will disappear and the smaller veins within the leg are now trying to reattach themselves to another bigger vein which is quite normal," he said. 'I am quite happy with your recovery but we need to keep monitoring you,' and with those parting words he said, "We'll see you tomorrow."

During the interview I heard a voice ask the nurse if the curtains could be opened as he felt claustrophobic. In response she said, "Sorry we cannot do anything until after the patient's interview." Then like a stage production with back lighting from the window, the curtains are drawn, and I gaze upon a new face occupying the bed next to me. The patient has yet to have his operation; he slides off his bed and introduces himself as Max. He tells me that he is not sure when he will have the big cut, but when he does he will be provided with a mechanical valve! He will be able to join the Fraternity of Clunk! Clunk!

Time flies and before we know it the evening food trolley arrives, laden with delicacies. My entrée commences with hot, piping chicken soup, three small spring rolls with a light, no-fat sauce; followed by steamed, local fish with a hint of fresh lemon and parsley herbs that lightly enfolds over it, and apple pie crumble with ice cream that will be washed down by a full bodied cup of coffee made from the very best of Brazilian coffee beans. Salivate if you would with me, but don't despair. My meal was a disaster, bland beyond words, however, I force myself to eat it but just a little crack pepper and a sprinkling of fresh lemon juice would have made a big difference to the taste of the fish. The things we dream of that are often close but so far away.

The creative thoughts within me have found a solution to my problem with the recliner. It is simple! I will leave the footrest down, move the extra chair closer to me, place a pillow on it and now I am independent. I can now raise my legs and rest them on the seat, push the chair away to lower them, and be able to stand, to visit the bathroom or go for a short walk. I no longer need to call the nurse for her assistance in getting up.

What a genius!

The window curtains are closed, and I decided to go for my short, shuffle walk before sleeping and to brush my teeth. The lights will be switched off soon and sleep is just around the corner; I am now comfortable in the recliner and I am covered with a thick, warm blanket. Pleasant dreams come to all who wait.

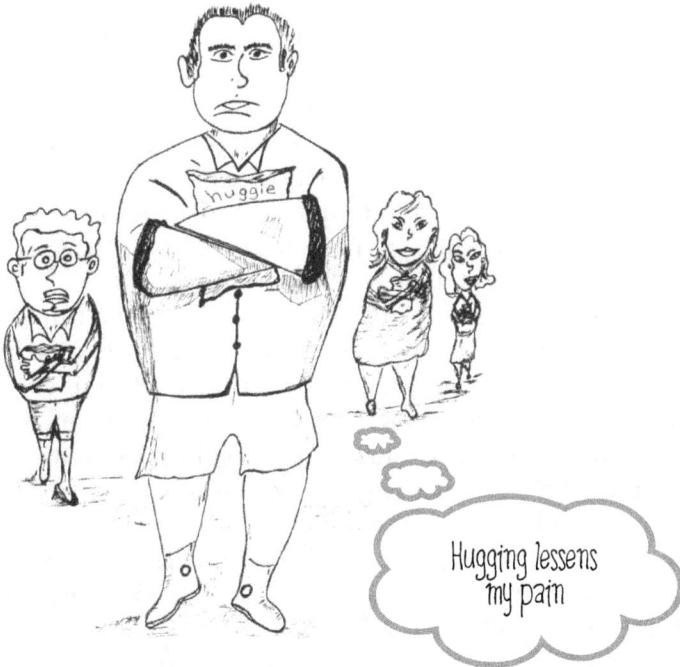

Chapter 18
Day 3 Post Op

What the...! I'm dreaming the dream of dreams, when they are shattered by a burst of overhead lights being switched on! In the early hours of the morn, voices are loud as they break the silence of those in slumber; curtains are drawn around the bed of an elderly patient! "What is your name?" "Where are you?" "What is the date of your birth?" A litany of questions is asked by the night nurse in order to test the mental state of the groaning person who is in obvious pain. What has happened? No doubt the grapevine will tell us.

Where once I was in dreamland, I groggily opened my eyes to the turbulence within the ward! I am now wide-awake and knowingly accept that sleep will be elusive and out of the question. Painkillers have been administered to the patient and his groans are now at a minimal, as the lights are switched off. The nurses once again go quietly about their business but not before issuing an apology for waking us up and a gentle request for us to go back to sleep. Ha!

What the...! I have just dozed off, I don't believe it! What's next, as I awake with a start? My heart is galloping like cattle in a stampede. Then it slows for a few seconds and begins again as if at a dance, but unable to decide whether it is a quickstep or a salsa! My hand wanders around the blanket for the call monitor until I finally grasp it, and press the button for the nurse. When she arrives I tell her the problem and she asks me to relax. What more can I do with a thumping heart but then I go into my relax mode to try and slow it down. The nurse has gone to phone to confer with the duty doctor who advises her to give me a tablet called Amiodarone that will regulate my heart rhythm. She should also monitor and record my heart beat intervals. After a while the heart seems to reach its normal beat and in a relaxed state, I am able to fall back to sleep thinking of *a tablet for you, a tablet for me, we then join hands and sing, We'll have a tablet for two.*

I have just managed a few hours sleep when lights are switched on once more, and as the curtains are drawn back across the window, the early dawn filters through the leaves of trees outside, into the ward. 'What is it this time?' I ponder and realize that a new day confronts us.

Before breakfast my first chore is to walk to the nurse's station to weigh myself, only to discover that it is hovering about the 73kgs, it is like the temperature in wintertime and falling! By the time I walk back to my bed the spirits have flown through the warm air and dropped clean pj's and towels onto my bed.

The bathroom is free and I move quickly to take possession of it, but not before I greet Max and Bill a "good morning." My facial bristles are about to sprout into a bush land setting, more-so that I have not shaved for four long days and it is time to regain my youthful looks of yesteryear! The TED stockings and the leg dressing were removed earlier so I take particular attention to ensure that the wound is washed clean without fear of giving birth to a bacterial baby! I am still wary of my unsteadiness during showering, however, when I finish, a new man walks out from the confines of the bathroom.

My breakfast awaits me as I approach my bed, although there is nothing special, I ensure that every morsel is eaten to help me regain some of my lost weight. Max has ordered porridge and he has smothered it with milk and honey, whilst Bill who is diagonally opposite me is enjoying his cornflakes.

Breakfast is over and the reds, browns, whites and pinks of the medication tablets face their downhill slide into the stomach once again. It is becoming monotonous but necessary! Although my blood pressure and pulse readings are continually monitored every four hours, the incident with my racing heart in the early hours of the morning requires me to have the pleasure of a one hour conversation with a delightful, young nurse who tells me, "I'm a charmer." She continues to monitor my heart beat whilst we talk about her goals and aspirations, then before we know it the hour is up and she returns to the nurse's station to write up my chart. Meanwhile, I look forward to the vampire who will fly into the ward later in the morning, to give me another love sting and to have a happy, informative conversation about her daily job.

Miguel, the male nurse who has worked the night shift, has asked me to move from the recliner to the bed because he needs to remove the all important pacing wire that hangs limply from my chest. He assures me that there is no pain; breathe in, hold, and pulls, the wire gracefully slides out from a minute puncture hole that he swabs and then covers it with a clean dressing. He tells me that I need to stay on the bed for at least an hour.

A young Fijian lass, who is studying nursing at the James Cook University in Townsville is in the ward to help and observe the work of the nurses. While being monitored, she swabs my leg wound with the orange-red betadine solution, places on a fresh sterile dressing then faces the task of pulling and tugging my TED stockings on. During this activity we talk about Fiji, her family and how long she has to study at the university. It was a warm and interesting conversation that both of us enjoyed.

After she leaves, I continue with my extraterrestrial breathing game with the apparatus and find it much easier to control and reach the required level. These daily breathing exercises are essential for a quick recovery and I usually do more than is needed, with the knowledge that without increasing my breathing capacity then my walking will suffer! The corridors await and I must soldier on!

How do I say it? My internal, river canals are facing a beaver-like dam and the all important tablets are not taking effect! I discreetly ask the nurse if there is a dam-busting bomb available, she eyes me and nods her head secretively and replies "don't go away, I'll be back!" A short time later she returns with 45mls of a clear solution in a measuring cup, she said, "drink this it will do wonders for you but be aware of its explosive nature!" I look at it, take a gentle smell, then gulp it down and ask, "What is it?" "Genlac," she replies as she walks away. True to her word, I hear the call of the wolves and I hasten to the bathroom, emerging later with largest of grins. Bill asks, "Did it work?" Like a Cheshire cat I point to my smile and nod with satisfaction. Bill calls for the nurse and said, "I want a dose of the same magic that you gave Loury." Walking back to my recliner, I remark, "Oh! What heavenly bliss!"

The delightful vampire arrives and with outstanding efficiency creates a small sting as she removes a small quantity of my life blood that is ensnared in a capsule destined for the pathology unit for testing. This is Medical science at its best.

Nela and Linda have arrived but their time is short. Linda has come to say how much she enjoyed her four weeks stay with us and so with a hug, a kiss and a fond farewell both leave for the Airport for Linda is to catch her return flight to Cairns and eventually back to Seattle via New Zealand. I was grateful for her time and appreciated her thoughtfulness and care.

Lunch bells are ringing and I sit down for a meal that is fit for a king, it is light, enjoyable repast that is followed by the fruit that caused the downfall of Adam! I ponder what my next meal will be; I know its curry and rice.

I'm on top of the world and when Dr Rajiv arrives with his entourage and with no disrespect I greet them with, "The Bollywood choir has arrived to sing a few songs of wisdom to me." They all laugh, the Doctor smiles and replied, "See I told you this is my model patient, he is always happy and smiling." Now you can compare him with others who are unhappy and their quest for 'why me' answers. 'Having asked the usual questions, they pull back the curtains, tell me to enjoy my dinner and depart the ward for their next patient.

The seconds have turned into minutes, then hours and after several short conversations with Max, Bill and his charming wife Elizabeth. We are surprised by the appearance of the dinner trolley with our sumptuous meal. I park myself on the edge of the bed, pull the bedside table towards me and lift the covers from the plates to reveal my curry and rice. I organize myself by buttering my cold, bread roll and tossing pepper over my dinner. My first mouthful proves a delight but it is not Nela's curry nor is it chili hot; needless to say that I did it justice, by mopping up the sauce residue and leaving the plate greasy clean. Red jelly and ice cream follows and I am visibly sated and gratified.

Max and I sit by the window sipping our coffee and watch two bush turkeys that have taken up residency in the trees outside. Max tells me that it brings back memories of his youthful days when he went camping with his dog and his horse, in the fog shrouded forests of the mountainous hillsides of New Zealand.

Darkness comes quickly, and the nurse draws the curtain across the window and for a short time, our reality TV excursions down memory lane comes to an end. We decide it's time for a walk along the corridor to help digest our food before we are called to the land of slumber.

Chapter 19
Day 4 Post Op

Reflections. I woke up without looking at my watch, and decided to have my shave before the others stirred and hastened to have their own ritual, morning ablutions. For some unknown reason I was feeling great, and upon leaving the bathroom I bumped into Miguel, the male nurse, who asked, "Do you always get up this early?" I looked at him mystified and in reply said, "Why, it's 6.00am and I can see the dawn filtering through the gaps in the curtains!" He laughed and said, "It's only 4.30am and it's the rays from the outside electric lights that you can see. 'What a numbskull,' thought. I should be sleeping and now I'm wide-awake! Back to my recliner to try and catch a few more ZZZ's, but they elude me, so I take the time to reflect on all that has happened.

Amidst all the questions of my emotions and feelings prior to and after the operation, I asked myself, 'what control did I have over them? Did I have enough information to base my control over them? My answer, 'none,' because at 72 I have maintained my philosophy of inner strength through the mantra of, *If I am not in control of things, I am not going to worry myself sick over them and build a monument of stress and tension in my body.*

Emotional questions that spring to mind are: How did I feel when I first learnt that I needed an aortic valve replacement and a triple by-pass? *Was I afraid? Was I anxious? Did I feel sad or depressed?* None of the above, believe it or not! Que sera, sera! What will be, will be! Although, flitting through my mind for a minute or two was the regret, that the family vacation trip to the Philippines had to be cancelled, it was a trip that everyone had been looking forward to, with the meeting of family and friends once more.

But then, did I sit down and immediately write letters to my loved ones and friends before the operation, because of the ugly questions that hover in the back of the mind and are brought to the forefront when one makes mountains out of molehills.

What if something goes wrong? What if the problem recurs several years down the track? What if I'm one of the 2% of patients that do not make it? What if I was not born? What if a helicopter fell on me after the operation? 'How many, what ifs do we need to take on board to make ourselves physically ill? I asked myself as I glanced at my watch. 'Why didn't I show any fear, anxiety, sadness or anger?' Did I repress these emotions within my body to re-emerge into some other dreadful disease later in life? Again, I answered no, otherwise I would have been reduced to a gibbering mess that would not have escaped either of my loved ones or friends.

'Nevertheless, how did I remain calm amongst all that was happening?' I pondered this question as I gazed at the overhead lights as if seeking an answer from their glow in answer to my enigma.

Firstly and simply, I acknowledge the fact that our holiday on earth will come to an end sometime, and that I have no control over the outcome, what-so-ever! So why worry about it?

Secondly, my inner calmness was achieved through 35 years of playing and coaching basketball, being involved in other sports, and reading numerous motivational books, all of which molded my character into lifelong experiences.

Lastly, studying the Filipino art of "Arnis" (stick) fighting and the Japanese martial art of Aikido and KI development, were the stepping stones in achieving how to get my One Point and extending my KI (energy), through the skills of learning proper breathing techniques. What the...?

If you watched the original movie "The Karate Kid," you would have seen the extension of KI in action. When the sensei clapped his hands together, closed his eyes to get his One Point, and then applied his hands to the painful areas of the shoulder and the thigh to extend his KI. All mumble jumble? No! Although limited to surface pain I have achieved good results by using it on injured basketball players and others.

Basically, it means to unify the mind and body, to achieve inner calmness. It is not difficult to achieve and everyone has the ability to learn it providing they have an open mind! (Chapter 27 - "How to achieve KI development")

I have been asked whether I had any hallucinations after the operation, but again I must answer, "None!" When I asked for the reasons behind the question, I was told that some patients suffer from a withdrawal of drugs and the aberrations in different forms that seem real and vivid, manifest themselves on the walls, such as spiders, waterfalls, fairy lights or colorful stripes. I was told that this was a normal occurrence. I thank the gods that I did not have this experience of illusions, although it may have sent me on a journey of discovery.

There is movement around the ward as the lights are switched on and curtains of privacy are withdrawn back. I decide to go for a couple of laps before taking the usual shower. On the way back, the nurse waylays me to quickly weigh myself; by this time my weight should be back to normal but alas I am still low at about 74kgs. I am not concerned as I needed to lose some body fat around my love handles.

Later in the morning, I will be attending a show and tell activity via a cardiac education session. The occupational therapist's talk should be interesting and informative as it will relate to my resumption of daily activities, return to work and learning how to conserve my energy. A social worker will later enter the scene to discuss our home situation, how to adjust with the coping and stress process that may occur from our emotional reactions after the operation. Time is on the move and my discharge from the hospital is eminent in the next week. So the powers to be, will be starting the administration wheels of paperwork to organize my farewell from the Cardiac Ward and the Townsville Hospital

In the meantime I will have a shower, dress my leg wound and replace the TED stockings. I continue using my breathing machine and working on my lap work around the corridors. I usually stop on the glass-covered walkway between buildings to soak up the sun that creeps over the roof tops into the children's playground and finally through the windows. What a joy it is to have the sun on your face and body! Unfortunately, I cannot stay too long as the legs become weary from standing.

My neighbour across the aisle from me had a bad night and was accusing the doctors of not giving him the correct medication. The tirade kept on for the rest of the morning. Later, he was obviously given a calming medication because he was seen by a bevy of doctors. He eventually went for an x-ray and had further blood tests on his frail body. We learnt later that he had a fall and the x-rays indicated that there was some pressure at the base of his skull and an operation seemed very likely the following day.

The dietitian has made an appearance to discuss the need to target a healthy lifestyle and from her interesting talks, we can reduce the risks of further heart disease by eating healthy, increasing physical activity, losing weight when needed, being less stressed, ensuring that medications are taken every day and giving up smoking. The latter can go down the drain, I cannot understand why people who smoke cigarettes want to make the tobacco companies and their directors rich, but that is my opinion! However, I must ask the question, 'Who controls whom?' However, a tip for the smokers, 'you will have to give up smoking at least 6 weeks before your pending surgery in order to give your lungs and heart a chance to improve. Ensure that you advise the surgeon and the anaesthetist that you 'smoke.'

Meanwhile, by perchance my love affair with delightful types of cheeses must either come to an end or limit my intake, because of the high risk of saturated fats. My eyes are teary as I think of the many, long years I have made toasted cheese sandwiches, eaten cheese with the sourness of green apples and now I must say a fond farewell to them. Fare thee well, oh, heavenly cheese.

I do not have to worry about my sodium intake because we use very little in our cooking and are very conscious of how much sodium is found in the food we purchase. On the other hand we ensure that our fibre consumption includes a range of vegetables, seeds, nuts, grains, cereals, wholemeal or grain bread and fruit in our daily diet. The all important eight glasses of water is also part of my daily regime when at home, because I believe it has helped in preventing or cutting down the incidents of gout and ridding my body of the toxins that are present in my medication.

The Dr Rajiv and his retinue share a brief stopover and he tells me that I should be going home in the next day or two, but this will depend upon further blood tests, x-ray and an ECG examination. I look forward to the day and wish them all a happy weekend.

The quietness of the ward is disrupted as the lunch trolley makes a noisy appearance as one wheel seems to be sticking. I lift the cover and inspect my garden salad and I am deeply surprised by the amount of green leaves, tomatoes, onions, radish and the three different types of meat that are heaped into the large, white bowl. A small sachet of mayonnaise, pepper and a buttered bread roll makes for a very delicious lunch.

For the first time I am able to read and concentrate on my paperback, so I settle comfortably in the recliner with my juice and a bottle of water readily handy on the bedside table. I ensure that I don't get too comfortable as I must make time to do a few laps and the use my breathing machine.

It is Saturday and through the day I have had visits from representatives of the different denominations, it was certainly thoughtful of them to take the time to see us and be able to have a chat no matter how brief their stay. It was also nice to see the number of Cook Islanders visiting Bill; I eventually discover that he is a Pastor of the Presbyterian Church. It is a quiet day and in the meantime Max and I have our usual conversations about New Zealand until the arrival of his daughter, son-in-law and his sister, Kush, who had just arrived from the home country that morning. Max will learn today when he will go for his aortic valve replacement; he has opted for a mechanical valve and so enters the Fraternity of Clunk! Clunk!

Nightfall is not too far away and after dinner, they say silence is golden but not here, you need activity to stop boredom from interfering with our recovery. Sunset gives way to the night sky, the curtains close on another day and the lights are switched off as the night shift takes over. What delights will they spring upon us during our hours of sleep! Goodnight!

Chapter 20
Day 5 Post Op

Heavenly Footsteps. Today will be like yesterday, except during the early hours of the morning, I sub-consciously awake with the sounds of wump! wump! From the rotors of the medical rescue helicopter hovering overhead. Yet, once more it brings another serious patient into the hospital.

Seeking the comfort of the blanket, I fall back into a deep sleep; but again like every other morning there is a burst of light, a rustle of curtains being drawn, that pulls me to the surface of consciousness. Saturday has rolled into Sunday, and the grey, leaden skies have beckoned the first rays of light to make an appearance, whilst from the surrounding hill a breeze blows down amongst the trees outside my window.

Lazily, I look around and notice very little movement from my fellow patients, until eyelids twitch and heads turn from side to side that indicate that my mates have decided to join me with a chorus of, 'Are you sleeping? How are you today?' I smile to myself and snuggle deeper into the blankets not wanting to make the first move! Knowingly, I will do the opposite and head for the bathroom. Alas, I stretch, yawn and head for my target. But…!

The ward nurse who is wide-awake notices the secretive patient tip-toeing across the room, waylaying me she said, "When you have finished preening yourself, I need you to gently stand on the scales and see whether you have gained some weight." I replied with another yawn, "okay."

True to my word and with her eagle eyes upon me, I leave the doorway of the bathroom and like a butterfly in motion I land on the designated scale. The digital numbers do not falter either one way or the other from yesterday's weigh-in! Like the famous quote of Muhammad Ali, "I float like a butterfly and sting like a bee!" I would have had my hands full in trying to hit my way out of a brown paper bag at my lost weight.

Just as I settle down in my nice, clean pj's onto my bed, the heavenly footsteps of the nurse approaches me once more! Feeling hemmed in I ponder the reasons for this sudden urge to speak to me. Is it my magical Paco Rabanne after shave, or the slim 6-pack that once assailed a trim body? Neither! She just wants to tell me that I will have a chest x-ray and an ECG after breakfast. *What is that tune?* I mused, 'A swish here! A swish there! A swish! A swish!" Makes the heart jingle, jangle whilst doing the skeleton rock!'

Breakfast comes and goes! I've made a few circuits around the centre block of the Ward. Then walk to the building crossover, to feel the sun energize every atom within my body that spreads rapidly creating a warm glow to a skin that has paled over the past few days.

My chauffer driven wheelchair rolls into the ward and although I feel fit to walk, hospital policy dictates that an orderly pushes me along the corridors, into the elevator, along another corridor to my destination. Half-an-hour wait and I gaze at the other patients who will also have the opportunity of becoming aliens for a brief time, as their bodies are bombarded and radiated with the minute atoms from the x-ray machine.

Later, I enter a darkened room with subdued lighting that creates a mystery of suspense until the young, female operator appears out of the gloom. We are separated by a thick, steel rail. She quietly explains what is to happen as electrodes are adhered to my skin. Then with her magic wand that is covered with a light coating of gel she slowly moves it over my chest. It is cold and it gives me goose pimples. I don't know who is more afraid, her or me? Tracking across my chest awakens the sonar.

She is about to hear the swish of my heart during the ECG examination. Should I break out in song? Before I can utter a word I hear swish, swish and her work begins. When finished she asks me to roll over onto my side so that she can play a tune on my muscular back. I've just had surgery and I've been sitting and sleeping on the recliner and now I've got to turn on my side which goes against sleeping on my back. I said, "I'll need your help to turn over as I have difficulty doing it by myself." I achieve the right pose, but grit my teeth trying to hold my body in check until the ordeal is over. When it does I find that my energy has been sapped and I have difficulty in claiming my position in the wheel chair once more.

Back to the ward, I have my usual blood pressure, pulse and temperature taken each morning only to have the same done all-over again later in the afternoon.

My nose twitches as it is assailed by the smell of a baked potato that wafts beyond the cover of my roast lamb and baked vegetable platter;

Lunch has arrived. Oh! What a delight! Oh! What joy! I attack it with relish and leave a greasy plate clean of juices! Then surrender to ice cream and apple pie! *What have I done to be granted this sumptuous feast?* I ask myself. It is simple just fill in the right square with your pencil, the night before. *What a moment of bliss* I sigh fully sated; coffee and a snifter of Tia Maria would go down nicely, but in your dreams! My lunch comes to an end.

Another bout with the cardiac educator and the occupational therapist, their supply of information is endless; however, it is necessary to remember the essential points that will help towards my recovery.

I traipse a light fandango and go on my merry way on a few circuits, before the arrival of my physiotherapist. Once more I hold in my gentle hands the machine of life as I continue with my breathing exercises. The importance of doing this exercise goes without saying; the lungs must show a continual improvement, even after being discharged and well into your walking fitness program. "Okay Loury, inhale a few rounds into your machine and see what level you have reached, and then we'll go for a walk," my physio said. She further says, "I have a surprise for you." as she ushers me towards and out of the fire exit door. There facing me is my freedom, the sun is shining and a slight breeze ruffles the leaves on the trees. Take some deep breaths and enjoy this short interlude. I can either go up or down but she has decided for me. "Let's go for walk upstairs." Dreading at walking a couple of floors of bending my knees I follow her to the first landing. Grinning she said, "Okay, let's head back to the ward, you've passed the test." I looked at her in amazement and said, "A test?" Wow!"

I continue to pay particular attention to the cleaning and dressing of my leg wound. However, the fun has begun with Nela's arrival and she faces the challenge to pull on my TED stockings. The nurse has given her a few tips of achieving this tricky maneuver to reach a smooth result. I think she will need to use the breathing machine herself as her energy has waned away. Of course, being a diabetic and having weak wrists does not help maintain her strength during these exertions. The nurse said, "Don't worry Nela you will get use to it!" Nela, in reply, grimaces!

Nela has met with several Filipino families and last night she attended a BBQ on the esplanade with them. She said it was cold but she wore a thick jacket to ward off the breeze coming in from the sea. Later on she attended a church service with Mary-Ann and her family and met a larger group of the Townsville Filipino community. Noting the time she needs to leave to catch the afternoon bus for the Hospital.

A light dinner arrives and I demolish it without fear of putting on weight. A cup of tepid tea washes down the last of my cold, bread roll but I am satisfied, especially when I look back to the days after my surgery where I had very little or no appetite at all. *Will it get any better at home?* I ponder, more so in the light of the dietician's information for healthy eating lecture.

Max, Bill and I have our after dinner conversation with much revolving around Max's turn under the gentle hands of the surgeon that is scheduled for Tuesday. Max does not want to take off his Maori amulet around his neck but realizes that it will get in the way of the surgeon. So he hopes that he will be able to wind it around his wrist before the operation.

A few turns of the corridors, a talk with the nurses, a look at the TV program in the small common room and my recliner bed lingers alone, calling me to its presence. I still find it easier to sleep in the recliner and be more independent in my movements.

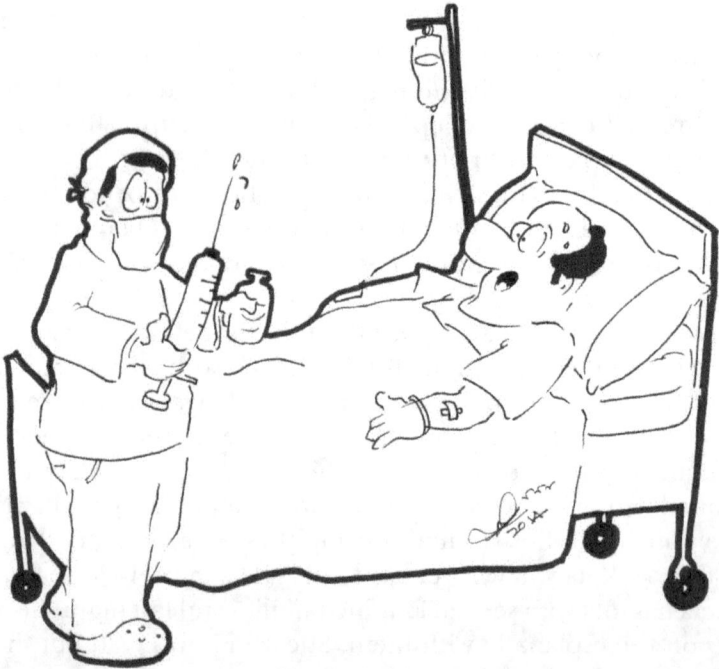

This won't hurt a bit! It's just a little pri.! Ooops! A sting.

Chapter 21
Day 6 Post Op

It's Happening! Had I walked through another time-warp or is this a dream? I watch the hot, desert sands form swirling eddies, as the strong winds blast across the archaeological site. The activity in the area is abuzz with muffled murmurs from the voices of the face covered workers. They are all waiting for the answers from radiation x-rays, the ECG and the blood tests, that were taken from the human form that was discovered in a small cave seven days ago and taken 9 kms to the camp hospital. They wonder how he came to be in the desert cave with very little water and a handful of nuts to ward off the hunger of a low fat diet? They wonder why he was strangely dressed; the archaeologists wonder if he had come through some sort of time-warp? The doctor has yet to arrive to give his approval for this human form to be released, so that he can return to the wilds of a city environment, but he too, will wonder about these anomalies.

Meanwhile, until his clinic review with the surgeon in six weeks time, the unruffled human continues to take the amiodarone tablet that regulates his heart rhythm. Likewise, the warfarin that has been prescribed continues its blood thinning act to treat and prevent blood clots forming around the new valve. Although they say that three is a crowd the medical profession thinks differently; iron supplements have recently been added to his diet of pills because a blood test indicated a low hemoglobin count. It's all happening! As the sands begin a dervish between the archaeological tents, he asks, "What next?"

The loose window shutters rattle and bang as the fierce desert winds continue their onslaught throughout the night. Suddenly, there is a lull in the wind gusts and the hospital staff can faintly hear an approaching ambulance from its wailing siren the sound of Yee! Yaa! They ready themselves and before long we are awakened from our deep stupor, as the lights are switched on. Doctors and nurses arrive wheeling in a groaning patient who consistently wails "don't touch me!" "I don't want that!" After sometime the patient yields to the calming medication and all of us fall back into fitful sleeps. Awakening next morning, we listen to the aggressive tones coming from the patient, who has decided to go out and smoke a cigarette even though he is still connected to his IV lines. This was against the specific wishes from the nurses and doctors. The patient said, "I'm going out for a smoke." Max and I look at each other and rolled our eyes, both of us asking the same question, 'Why does he want medical help?' *Put him at the end of the queue,* I mused.

Wearing a head scarf to protect her hair from the desert winds the pharmacist arrives to give her expertise and advice concerning the nine discharge tablets that I am presently taking. Her information includes the name of the tablet, brand name, what they are used for, the directions and a daily timetable as to when they should be taken. After I leave the hospital I will clutch in my hands a small plastic bag containing five days supply of tablets, but the tablets not on my discharge list are to be safely thrown away. Perhaps, if they were M & M's we could have a chocolate covered tablet party amongst the ruins of the desert rocks and buildings!

The temperature was extremely high as the doctor and his entourage battled their way against the hot desert winds to the hospital. Finally, they reach the steps. The threshold is thickly covered with a layer of crystal-like sand particles. They shake their clothes, but the fine sand has reached every nook and cranny of their attire. Walking into the ward, the doctor said, "I'm sorry but you will need to extend your stay with us for one or two more nights, because your blood test has indicated that your hemoglobin level is low. We will need another blood test today to ensure that you have a safe level before we can release you." Well! Murphy's Law has reared its ugly head once more, but I'm not in control so I'm not going to worry, and will take everything day by day. Who knows it might even be lower tomorrow.

The desert winds have abated and all is back to normal, and through the window I can see the distant mountains coming into view as the dust settles over the dunes that have moved yet again. The temperature will obviously soar, but the ward will remain cool as the generators that feed the air conditioning system units continue to chug along.

Before my low fat diet lunch appears, I wander over to the nurse's station to have my weight taken. It has dropped and I weigh 74.5 kgs. Any lighter and I'll be like a feather and take flight in the updrafts of the light desert air. However, lunch comes and goes, it is nothing to rave on about, but it is nourishing.

After lunch my pleasant vampire flies in for a few grams of my precious red blood. *Anything for science and my well-being,* muse as the needle hovers over the pores of my skin, and like a submarine, dives into the shallows of my arm searching for that ever thin vein. Eureka! Touch down! The gentle hand of the nurse withdraws the rich, cerise claret into the vial of the syringe. I receive a white cotton ball to press over the tinniest of openings for a few seconds; this is to ensure that the drops of gold do not become a miniature underwater, seamount volcano! Finally, an antiseptic band aid is applied with tender care.

The thin, snakelike scar that travels from above my knee to my ankle is healing quite well and hopefully, it will continue to do so! Another coating of the orange betadine solution is spread over it and a large sterile band aid ensures that infection does not become an unwanted visitor. Pondering over the scar, I think to myself, *If only it had been a large letter 'Z'.* I could have said, "Zorro had performed the surgery." I still need help in pulling on the TED stockings, but white does become me.

An attractive woman, enters my field of vision, and introduces herself as the community assistance officer. She explains her role and provides us with telephone numbers and names to contact when we returned to Cairns. We intend seeking their input, especially the occupational therapist, who will give us ideas about the installation of holding bars and shower extensions in the bathroom.

Night has fast approached; dinner has been masticated into fine sediments of food particles that are followed by the usual tepid cup of tea. It is still too early to sleep; a few circuits around the ward, and I wonder if a pedometer that measured our steps would have been a strong motivator in getting patients up and about more quickly. I think it would have certainly helped in providing an achievable goal. Food for thought!

Back to my lonely recliner, to read a little, then close my eyes to try to recapture my desert adventure. It's all happening, I reflect, as I pull the white, lightweight blanket over me.

Chapter 22
Day 7 Post Op

The Winner is? Lights on, curtains drawn, It's just after 6.00am; I thrash around, sink down, eyes open, eyes closed, for a moment, then back to the surface and into reality.

No desert storms, no archaeological sites, no dinosaurs, just a couple of bush turkeys roosting in the tree outside my window. The darkness has faded, and there is a glint of sunshine as the sun rays filter through a few clouds and then penetrate the leaves of the trees outside the window, *'It's going to be a great day if I get the all clear to leave the sanctuary of the hospital,'* I mused.

"Well is this going to be the day? Will I change out of my hospital pj's for the last time, to get dressed into a more comfortable shirt and shorts? Rather than trying to bend over and tie shoe laces, or to get Nela to tie them for me, I have bought a new pair of sandals. Will this be an occasion to remember or will I need to stay another day?" I asked myself.

Heading for my daily preening, I commandeer the bathroom, after having first removed the dressing from my leg wound *Will I get my Purple Heart medal for the scar*, I ponder.? Back into the ward, feeling like a new man, there is pep in my step. I look for Max, but he has disappeared behind a wall of curtains, that emanate the sounds of bumble bees buzzing around their hives. He is having his full, manly, body shave. Yes! This is his day! He will become a member of the mechanical valve fraternity of clunk! Clunk! Much later he is wheeled out of the ward, to "our best wishes and good luck."

The breakfast trolley silently arrives in the ward. This a new trolley or have they fixed the wheels? Quietly, the orderly distributes our tray of treats! My tray offers cereal, a cold bread roll, milk, juice, butter, jam and two sachets of coffee. This will provide my morning sustenance until the gnawing of my insides tells me that lunch is just around the corner!

I enjoy the quiet solitude of breakfast, while looking out of my window at people passing by. They come in all shapes and sizes, wearing

78

dark winter attire, as it seems' quite breezy outside. I try to envisage by their clothing what each person does. What they may have had for breakfast, how they came to the hospital and why some meet with friends or colleagues and converse for a short time, and then they meander down the concrete path. Others have young children in tow, some young, others older; while others walk hurriedly along sipping a hot coffee, while a discarded coffee cup is carried by the wind into the bushes beyond.

Breakfast is over, and I do my own circuits of the ward and stop on the building cross-over as usual to catch some sunshine that beams between the two brick buildings. Shining on my face, I feel the sun shooting energy through my whole body. I'm on top of the world!

Back in the ward and the nurse tells me that I have a good chance of being discharged sometime after lunch. I feel elated and will contact Nela by mobile as soon as it is confirmed. Yippee! It seems the winner is…!

It is really happening! I am given an appointment letter to see Dr Tam in six weeks time in Townsville. He will assess my well-being, and check to see if I have any problems related to the surgery, importantly, he will also give me the all clear to drive my vehicle. We often take things for granted, but we are at a loss when we cannot get behind the wheel of our car! If you do decide to drive a car before this approval is given and you have an accident, then you may not be covered by your insurance! The main problem is that you may damage your sternum because of the stress you put on it while steering! Do you really want another operation?

Another discharge letter will also be given to me to take to my GP who will assess the level of the warfarin that I am taking. Thankfully, I will be taken off the warfarin after the six weeks, but I will continue to take the 100mg of aspirin that will also do the work of thinning my blood.

My celebratory lunch has arrived and I munch like a rabbit through a tossed salad of green leaves strewn with a sachet of vinaigrette, and devour the three different slices of thick meat that adorns the pile of leaves. This is washed down with a packet of orange juice, followed by my wholesome banana; butter and jam bread roll and washed down with a much warmer cup of tea. Like a rocket I am all fuelled up ready for the blast-off! Start the count down.

Shortly after lunch, the travel officer arrives and hands me the documents for our 5.00pm return flight to Cairns. Immediately, I call Nela to be at the hospital before 2.30pm as the ward nurse now confirms that I would be leaving about 3.30pm.

Hastily, I put things into my carry bag, but have to wait to complete this chore until the pharmacist hands me a treasure trove of different coloured pills that will last me five days. Thereafter, I need to see my GP for more! Packing my bag was easy, as my weeks supply of pj's I had brought with me were still in their zip lock bags. I'll miss the long, loose, airy hospital pj's that showed the world my athletic slim body to the hospital populace!

Dr Rajiv has just popped in to tell me that my hemoglobin level was okay and that he had given his approval for my discharge. I thanked him for his medical skills and his ability to work wonderful miracles with Dr Tam and the team. He wished me a safe journey home, a successful recovery and a long life!

I recognize that my recovery after the operation was due to a complete team effort that included the surgeons, nurses, the fabulous vampires, the physiotherapist and other medical professionals who I would not be able to name the list is vast. However, it would be remiss of me if I did not recall Amy, Clare, Kiara, Margaret, Meg, Louise and Miguel; a fine group of dedicated young people who have given their lifetime energies into caring for others. I know some are continuing their studies through the Townsville Bible College, and I wish them well in their endeavors and success for the future. To those names that I have forgotten, my apologies, but you know who you are and from Nela and I, a very big thank you and keep on smiling. If you are feeling down, just remember you made a 72 year old Adonis, feel 21 again with your energy, wit, smiles and laughter.

Nela has arrived with two carry-on wheelie cases. She realized that I would not be able to carry my bag, hence the clothing chariots. Alas! I now have to unpack my bag and put the contents into my modern chariot. Just as I started, the pharmacist arrives with my bag of discharge medication tablets and gives me some last minute instructions.

Having changed earlier into my going home attire, I made my way around the nurse's station saying my farewells; a few receive my special hugs, especially "Canada," a Canadian nurse who was working her way around Australia; also to Bill and Elizabeth who were still waiting for a prognosis concerning another problem with him.

The nurses do a tremendous job, and this is one of the reasons why I needed to become more independent, rather than be dependent on them. More-so when they are busy with other patients and no matter how many times you try to buzz them they are often delayed in answering your call. This causes frustration in the mind-set! It must be remembered that other patients may be in more pain than you. However, the old adage of, "you cannot please some of the people all of the time," is true! We can be more appreciative of their time for these fabulous angels. Importantly we must remember that we made the choice to have the operation, and we are alive! With that in mind, I don't intend to spiral downwards, whatever the situation! Spiraling upwards like a huge twister will turn those small steps of recovery into giant ones!

Although I was feeling okay all the emotion has drained some of that pent-up energy and I wasn't sure how far I could walk upon leaving the hospital. More-so of the slight dip in my hemoglobin level two days ago. My thoughts must have followed the ESP waves to the nurse's station, and before I knew it an orderly arrived with a wheelchair for my immediate transport to the hospital bus. I was pushed along the well lit corridors to the elevator, and along several more for the last time, to the double doors that opened into the car park. Travelling along the main road to the airport, I felt as if I was in a time zone as vehicles of all sizes and colours whizzed past our eight seater bus. Amazingly I felt free after my nine day stint in the hospital and I reflect back on those first days with assorted lines attached to my body.

We finally reach the airport and I clumsily alight to help Nela with the bags, but the driver was well ahead of us and had everything under control as he took us to the check-in counter. We received our boarding passes and the customer service officer asked, "Do you need a wheelchair?" In reply, I whispered, "yes, please!" "We will have one standing-by when we start boarding because it is a fair distance for you to walk to the plane," he said.

We still had some time to wait and I was famished with all the exertion, so we ordered cappuccinos and two toasted ham and tomato sandwiches, and thought we were in for a nice treat. Not so! The coffee was tepid, the sandwiches were bland, but we could not blame the seller too much a she was inundated with passengers ordering similar snacks. Finishing, I wander over to the news stand and staring at me with weeping eyes was my favourite double dipped chocolate 'cherry ripe!' I did not waver, and looked longingly at something I dare not have...... for the moment!

Our flight is called, and I am wheeled along the safety fence to our waiting aircraft, and find that I am the last to board. I am visibly surprised, when I am asked to stand in a cage and holding on to the rails, the mechanical machine elevates me level to the floor of the plane, where I step into it with ease, only to be confronted by the stares of my fellow passengers, who wonder, "What's wrong with him?" Fifteen minutes later we rumble down the tarmac and lift-off into a clear blue sky... Destination Cairns!

Chapter 23
Recovery

A New Journey. The flight home is uneventful. Nevertheless, as the sun sets over the horizon, we look in wonder at the high level of cirrus clouds that are filled with a kaleidoscope of colours ranging from the reds, oranges, mauve, to pink and to other hues. Just below us the dark greens of the rainforest unfolds before our eyes as dusk begins to wane, but not before the mind conjures the existence of the animals, plant life and the insects within its natural environment.

Then the plane begins its descent, and we look upon the turbulent nature of the landscape, when millions of years ago, volcanic eruptions and earthquakes unleashed powerful pressures on the land to create uplifts, faults and folds over the earth's surface. This further created mountain ranges, gorges, lakes, rivers that flowed between towering cliffs, and layer upon layer of earth covered villages, towns and cities of old. Life is worth living, I reflect, as I tighten my seat belt and smile at Nela.

Before us the lights of the airstrip, blink their welcome. Bleeding off speed and decreasing altitude, the pilot lines up the runway, gliding down the tyres gently kiss the surface of the tarmac to make a perfect landing as a curtain of darkness envelopes us. The reflection of the lights from the terminal buildings shimmer on the darkened tarmac as the aircraft comes to a halt and the engines are shut down for the night.

It is quiet except for the passengers shuffling about taking their possessions from the overhead lockers and moving forward to disembark. There is a lull in the movement and I stand, but there are others following on, so I wave them forward, not wanting to hold them back!

I gingerly walk down the four wobbly steps to the ground. The hostess informs us that a buggy was going to collect us. It felt like an eternity and we were just about to give up and walk to the terminal because the wind had turned bitterly cold. The prospect of catching the flu was not on my agenda! Then from out of the gloom, we are silhouetted against the aircraft by two shining bright eyes that quietly approach us and then stop beside us, our transport has arrived. In a few minutes we reach the warmth of the terminal, collect our bags and amble off to the taxi stand.

Home at last! What a sight! Darren and Danni have left the lights burning and we are not totally in the dark, when fumbling around with the key and trying to put it into the lock. We open the door and look in wonder, as we step inside and familiar surroundings unfold before our eyes. *One journey has ended and another is to begin,* I ruminate as I slowly wheeled the chariots of clothing to the bedroom to unpack.

Both Darren and Danni have worked their culinary skills, in preparing a light meal of tossed salad, covered with slivers of sliced chicken and cashew nuts together with fresh, crusty, wholemeal bread. A delicious mixture of fresh fruit and berry yoghurt for our dessert tops off our meal. The one thing missing was a bottle of nicely chilled Marlborough sauvignon blanc wine. Yet I am ever conscious of the dreaded gout and the excruciating pain that prevails within the body. I err on the side of caution!

I've decided to sleep on the recliner for the first night, but that proved to be a mistake! The hospital recliner was more upright, whereas I was continually slipping downwards on mine and this put added pressure on my sternum and caused discomfit! Nevertheless, I persisted and had a fitful sleep; my restlessness was further exacerbated by my desire to visit the royal chambers throughout the night.

Dawn is beginning to break, and I listen pleasantly to the birds twittering amongst the trees outside. I watch with interest as two birds fight amongst themselves, and I wonder why so early, but recognize that they are being playful with each other.

My first day at home and it has just turned 6.30am, and I'm ready to hit the floor running, but, alas! Although I want to get up, I find it difficult once again to push the recliner foot rest down and need Nela's helping hand. But I need to wait for Nela to complete her yoga exercises, this does not stop me from taking off my TED stockings and removing the leg wound dressing with some degree of difficulty. I have to get back to that independence I had during my stay in hospital.

Finally I head for the shower, but realize that it is not as large as the hospital bathroom, and more importantly it does not have any grab bars installed. A plastic chair is required so that I can sit down, rather than slipping and sliding in an old time telephone box. Safety is now a very important issue! I call Nela for her assistance and she duly arrives with a chair that is placed in the shower stall.

It is the first time that she has seen me in my birthday suit, and she is visibly, dismayed at my weight loss, exclaiming! "Look at your thighs! Where has all your muscle gone?" In reply, I said, "you're worried about my thighs, but where is my backside, it too has wasted away!" Looking at my image in the mirror, I shudder at the sight of another space alien who has suffered muscle meltdown.

Nevertheless, a hot shower, and a quick glide over my face with my Gillette mach 3 turbo razor heralds a burst of sustainable, energetic stamina that will help me throughout the day. Then out to the kitchen to partake of my usual dosage cup of medicated rainbow tablets that will ward off hidden gremlins within my body. Reflecting on my weight loss I start the morning breakfast with a bowl of muesli, fresh fruit, a good sprinkling of L.S.A. and linseed mix, with a wholegrain vitabrit swimming in a lake of milk. 'Operation Recovery' has began as I put spoon to cereal.

While eating on the patio, I focus my mind on a few jobs that needed to be done before the operation, but have now lapsed into a state of "sometime?" It will be great to actually do some light work around the house if I can, famous last thoughts, ha! However, I now have the responsibility to ensure that my health comes before other activities. Especially when trying to lift things around the house.

I will need to reread all the 'do's' and don'ts' from the Townsville Hospital cardiac services booklet that provides me with valuable information. I do not relish the thought of undue problems occurring because of my stupidity and having to face another operation to repair possible damage to my sternum. Furthermore, I do not want to put added pressure on the shoulders of Nela who is now my Carer.

I've been cut open, had surgery, appeared as a sick alien and now look towards the process of healing and taking care of my breastbone like a new born baby. My thinking cap will be on and must question every activity more-so if I feel any discomfort or I'm in cloud nine because of dizziness or shortness of breath. I still need to carry and use my huggie pillow whenever coughing or sneezing and for the next six to eight weeks. I will not be able to drive, in case complications occur during this time. What a bummer!

Even carrying shopping bags, if they weigh less than five kilos, good and well, but anything over that is a no-no! However, as the months flash past, I'll gradually be able to increase the load through my shoulders, nevertheless carrying bags of swimming salt and a heavy container of liquid chlorine is definitely out of the question. Fortunately, great friends are ready to provide that helping hand. Still, should my breastbone decide to dance a Spanish flamenco because of a clicking or movement sensation, then I may have hit a minefield of trouble. This is not going to happen!

The pressure of not being able to do the normal household chores is limited to light duties for the first two to four weeks. This no doubt, pleases Nela who now realizes that I need to avoid mopping, sweeping or vacuuming for about three months. Mowing is out of the question also because of the need to pull the starter cord! I'll really need to sit down with Nela and plan our attack on the minor problems ahead of us. Nevertheless, the important factor is to keep myself active within my energy capacity by pacing myself throughout the day.

Although I have had an aortic valve replacement and the triple by-pass, I should be wary of still catching an unwanted infection that develops into bacterial endocarditis or an infection of the heart valve and the surrounding tissue.

If you think of yourself as a space alien coming to earth, and due to a different atmospheric environment, an infection starts within in your body. Then from the outset the first port of call, for this infection to take place, is your mouth. Inflammation of the gums and teeth will create a problem, and allows bacteria to dive into the bloodstream to travel throughout the body and arteries, where it attaches itself around your newly placed heart valve.

Since the alien has come in peace, we ensure that he has been given antibiotic preventative medication prior to the operation. However, if a problem does occur after surgery, and red, open sores, oozing with toxins appear and show no sign of healing, or if there is a loss of appetite, sweating or fever then the old adage cries out, "the problem persists, see your doctor."

Fortunately, our space alien has the strength to push a button and from outer space an ever-increasing light grows bigger with intensity, until it hovers overhead and whisks him away into the midnight sky. But for us mortals we need to be vigilant with our health after surgery.

I can honestly say that this human alien did not suffer an emotional crisis that caused shock, anger, denial, anxiousness or depression, nor did I have any fear of death, anxiety or confusion. Upon reflection, I often ponder that question, but that is for the gods to answer. However, I do believe my years of deep breathing exercises contributed much to my inner calmness.

Nevertheless, as a former teacher, I constantly remind myself that each of us have individual differences that define our character. The sudden knowledge of our cardiac problem and the pending surgery, results in our mind having a wide variety of reactions that introduce the emotional crisis and stress within us. It only takes a word, a sentence that plants a seed that festers into a picture, a scene that puts us on the road to a roller coaster ride in our minds! What if..!

Love, care, communication and the necessity of seeking professional help or talking things over with your loved one or a friend, will greatly help towards overcoming the distress that you may encounter because of the sudden changes in your lifestyle and that of your carer.

Nela calls out, "Get yourself organized, it's 9.30 and we have the doctor's appointment at 10.30am!" Breakfast is over, dishes are washed and "I'm ready," I call out a little later as I comb the little hair I own over my skull.

Well it doesn't take long before I wish I could drive now rather than in six weeks time, as I pay the taxi driver the fare that has risen over the years. My mind begins calculations and comes to the final conclusion, at this rate we'll be singing on the corner for our taxi fares! Getting in and out of the taxi was an interesting activity that took away some of my energy.

Walking into Dr Brodie's surgery, I felt as if I was going on safari and all I needed to coordinate my white TED stockings and shorts was a pith helmet and a shot gun. Then emerging from the jungle of trees, and the tall savannah grass, a voice said, "Dr Livingstone, I presume?" But instead I heard a voice exclaim, "My god! Loury! You have certainly lost some weight," the receptionist said, as she checked off my name on her computer. Jokingly I said, "This is what happens when you go into hospital visibly fit and come out physically sick!"

Dr Brodie voices similar comments and since I am taking warfarin, he sends me down to the nurse to check out the INR (International Normalized Ratio) levels. Way over my head, still it made sense to the nurse, who said it was okay. Back to see the doc and we go over the results of the operation and my recovery needs. Another appointment for tomorrow to recheck the INR's once again. *This is going to be a tedious activity*, I mused thinking of the taxi expenses.

Home again, and I go for my short walk of ten minute periods, but my first obstacle is that I only have 100 metres of level roadway before I am faced with gradual inclines in all directions. This will suffice for the time being but as my strength and stamina increases so will my walking, then it will be downhill and uphill trips accompanied with my bottle of water to wade-off possible dehydration.

It is a nice day so I move my chair into the sun and remove my shirt to take in the vitamin D that the rays emit and begin reading my book. I've decided to move from the recliner to the guest room and will organize the bed later. Since I have had the double operation, I must sleep on my back for the next six weeks, wow! This is going to be a torturous, sleeping activity! However, with Nela's help we place as many pillows on it to make it comfortable and to ensure that I can sleep at about 45 degrees; this will also allow me to swing my legs off the bed, to be able to stand and to walk around, becoming more independent is a necessity, without causing undue stress on myself or Nela.

I feel like goldilocks and the three bears! Who's being sleeping in my bed? Well my sleep is continually broken by nature and I find that the softness of the mattress caused a sinking sensation that left me floundering and feeling the pressure on my sternum. It's only the second night, so I'll persist with it over the weekend to see if I can improve my sleeping posture.

It's Friday and another visit to the doctor is but hours away. I've taken my tablets, eaten breakfast, done my stretching, exercised my neck, arms and trunk, and then gone for my short walk, ensuring that my posture is good and that I walk tall! My daily walking program will improve my fitness; and especially, the muscle tone and strength that I had lost will gradually improve and return. It is a good way for me to practice my deep breathing exercises and extending my KI that strengthens my inner calmness.

I continually do my breathing exercises with the voldyne apparatus and ensure that my legs are elevated when I am reading for a long time. I limit my time on the computer. Of course, there is the constant need to use the 1-2-3 movement when rising and not using my hands for pushing up for support otherwise there is undue stress on the sternum.

A phone call from the Westcourt Community Health Centre has advised that a nurse will be calling on me next week to look at my chest and leg wounds and to offer nutritional and occupational therapy suggestions that will help the changes in my lifestyle.

Our neighbours of 22 years, Sue and Gary Schofield have come over to see me, and to offer their help in transporting me to the doctors or taking Nela shopping. This is what friendship is all about and we have no hesitation in accepting their generous offer. More-so, as we were due to go for my doctor's appointment within the hour.

Slumber comes easily, but I'm no Rip Van Winkle and with the shifting of the pillows, the continual hourly call to nature, and I become wide awake if I switch on the bedroom lights. So I tend to crash into the walls of darkness but the lack of a working flashlight does not help my cause of walking around being invisible. Fitful sleep becomes inevitable. Tomorrow is Saturday and I wonder what sports program will be shown on the telly.

Chapter 24
War of Attrition

Exhaustion. It is Saturday 15 May 2009. It had rained the night before and as I begin my walk, the awakening sunlight creates a glistening roadway triggering a figment of my imagination that transports me back into time, to the year 1800.

The droplets on the leaves have been transformed into hundreds of stalactites that hang from the ceiling of a huge, cold, misty deep cavern and from the floor stand the stalagmites that have grown from a similar source over hundreds of years. It is miserably cold and damp, yet hundreds of soldiers who have taken up residency huddle together to keep warm and try to sleep amid the small fires that dot the cave; others have taken refuge in smaller caves but the majority try to withstand the cold, yet shiver in their tents that litter the mountainside tracks.

The backdrop of fires cast deep shadows on the walls and the ceiling as a lone figure wrapped in a heavy greatcoat walks amongst his men, stopping occasionally to talk to them and to give them encouragement for the hardships ahead of them. He turns his head at the sound of hooves clipping the hardened surface of the cave floor. He walks over to a magnificent warhorse of Arabian origin that enjoyed flying over the desert sands and not floundering over ice-capped, craggy rocks of the Pennine Alps. Whispering softly into its ear while stroking its head he said, "Easy Styria, we will soon reach our destination and you will be able to run swiftly over the lightly covered fields of snow."

Now and then cold wind gusts invade the security of their temporary home. Looking out through the entrance the General gazes upon the steep foreboding mountain sides that his army must endure to conquer, if he is to cross through the Great St. Bernard Pass that is situated between the boundaries of France, Italy and Switzerland. Incensed that Austria had taken over an Italian territory that was annexed to France, he formed an army of 40,000 strong and left the undulating fields of France for the cragginess of the mountains that are the Pennine Alps to fight yet another battle for France.

I imagine the hardship of manhandling his heavy artillery pieces and supply wagons over the treacherous terrain; of his army experiencing tremendous ordeals of below zero temperatures, dangerous, snow filled crevasses, hidden rifts and walls of deep snow. My mind takes in the perilous and horrifying sights of nature that create the avalanches as a whole mountainsides collapse and slide downhill taking all before it.

Finally, once over the Alps his army advances to the Po valley in northern Italy where he surprises and defeats the Austrians at the Battle of Marengo. Although it was not all smooth sailing, he made an unusual military blunder and was nearly defeated. Likewise the Austrian General Michael von Melas suffering from injuries and thinking he had won the battle turned over control to a subordinate who was no match to ward off a brilliant counterattack that turned the battle into a famous French victory. The French General, also known as the le Petit Caporal (the little corporal) was reportedly the greatest military genius of his time and indeed probably the greatest general in history, the man, they called Napoleon Bonaparte. (From Wikepedia – the Free Encyclopedia - Napoleon Bonaparte/ Battle of Marngo/Michael von Melas/Austrian General).

So what has that got to do with my journey? I think of the their hardships, the logistical nightmare of moving 40,000 soldiers through treacherous terrains, their lack of winter clothing, food, water, firewood, feed for the animals etc. More importantly their lack of medical knowledge to what it is today. What kind of doctors and medicine did they have at their disposal? How did they maintain their positive attitude? What motivated them? Then I think of the present day of the stresses that we encounter and how they are overcome! How do we turn our problems into victories?

Then I am quickly shaken out of my reverie as a car horn blows, looking up I wave to the driver. I have increased my walk to fifteen minutes up and down the 100 metre roadway. I can probably walk longer but will follow the rules of not overtaxing my body to do more and using up vital energy and return home.

Breakfast is over and I do the things that need to be done. Then I move outside to do some sunbathing and use vitamin E oil over my wounds to improve the healing of the scar tissue. My book, a coffee and I settle myself into a comfy chair to read in the sunshine.

An uneventful morning and I move into the family room to watch the afternoon AFL football match where I doze. About 5:00pm in the afternoon, I feel something is not right, I'm feeling lightheaded and slight dizziness has put me into a brief spin. I ask Nela to take my blood pressure which is low but I decided to wait 30 minutes to see if there is a change. I am not suffering any pain, yet my heart is starting to jump around. I tell her, "You better call triple 000 because I am really not feeling too well."

She makes the call and speaks to the operator then answers a few questions. She tells me that the person on the other end needs to speak to me. I've slumped into the recliner and slowly get up and shuffle to the phone. I can barely whisper my replies to the questions asked of me. I am told that a paramedic is on the way. Handing the phone back to Nela I make my shuffling return to the chair, sink down and close my eyes.

About 5 to 10 minutes later a female paramedic arrives and introduces herself. Having asked the inevitable questions and taking my blood pressure she notifies her home base to send out an ambulance. Night has fallen and I am aware of the flashing lights that originate from the parked ambulance that whisks me to the Cairns Base Hospital Emergency Unit.

Wheeled into the unit I am moved from the ambulance gurney onto a hospital bed, where I face a bevy of doctors and nurses asking all the important questions that will narrow down my health problem. My blood pressure is taken every half hour and of course, the inevitable vampire seeks my bodily blood for tests to see if the problem lies in that area, whilst a little later I face the radiation of an x-ray machine. The results of the blood test have been assessed and a low haemoglobin level has been detected; immediately I am given one of two units of blood transfused to raise the count to an acceptable level. A doctor has advised me that I will be admitted into the hospital for an overnight stay, this information allays Nela, Darren and Danni's fears so they take their leave and go home.

Meanwhile, I continue to watch the non-stop activity of doctors, nurses and orderlies moving to and fro, as new patients arrive to go through a similar amount of medical checks. Some are quiet but others are in pain as indicated by their groans, whimper or moans. I am impressed by the efficiency of the staff and their workmanlike attitude in attending to patients. For some patients it is not enough and they want immediate attention and quick results, they forget or have no idea that assessments need to be accurate, to enable the doctors to make diagnostic decisions for the betterment of their health!

It is 10.56pm and an orderly arrives and I find myself wheeled through the emergency ward, with other patients eyeing my progress and wondering where I am headed. The corridors are well lit, and I survive the elevator ride to the 3rd floor. The castor wheels of the bed rotate quietly as I arrive without fanfare to Med 3 and moved to a vacant spot, where I am greeted by cardiac nurse Anita Basu.

The night passes quickly without any unforeseen dilemma's, yet by 7.30am the vampire arrives to take a further blood test from a well punctured vein, that results in winning a second unit of blood. It is certainly amazing how the human body heals itself! The doctors arrive to tell me that I can leave the hospital after lunch and further advise that I can stop taking the amiodarone tablet that regulates my heart rhythm and that the irbestaten tablet can be halved for my daily ration.

This is good news! So I contact Nela to pick me up. She arrives with young Sharleen Percali whilst her mother, Marietta finds a vacant car park. I am still weak in the legs and request a wheel chair to help me to the main entrance of the hospital. Home again, and I need to organize my walking schedule as this problem caused a minor setback in my recovery. Although I felt slightly exhausted by the drop in my haemoglobin level I was looking forward to building my stamina via the daily walks.

Nela has relegated herself to the guest room, while I take up residency in the main bedroom because of the on-suite situation. All the pillows have been moved and placed into position for my maximum benefit. Then sleep overtakes me. I woke up early without any premonition of what lies ahead of me and that will further slow a quick recovery.

Monday rolls into Tuesday and upon wakening I know that the gremlins have struck with full force. I am unable to move let alone trying to get out of bed, both feet and ankles are throbbing and I know that my gout has reared its ugly head. I call Nela and tell her the wonderful news; she is dismayed! The pressure of standing is excruciatingly painful, as my mind fleeting feels for Napoleon's soldiers fighting frostbite and the like on the Pennine Alps. But I'm not climbing the mountains, nor am I facing cold blizzards; is my pain any worst than theirs? I wonder in thought. Needless to say, both of us ask the same question, 'What has triggered the gout? What did I eat? Was it something in the blood ' transfusions' No matter how many questions we ask, the fact remains, 'I have gout and what do I need to do' I ponder, as I ask Nela to get the colchicine tablets that will combat this painful gremlin!

During the week, the pain eases in both feet and I am able to hobble to the bathroom by the weekend, but I still have to contend with waking up every two hours to relieve myself. The sticky, sinus discharge that gums up my mouth during the night also causes me to gargle and rinse out my mouth. Nela is doing a sterling job as my carer, but unfortunately, disaster strikes towards the weekend!

Gary and Sue Schofield have been outstanding in helping with transport since our arrival back from Townsville. We are about to embark on yet another visit to the doctor. But on this particular day, Nela has unwittingly stood on a palm nut, and twists her knee; before we know it she has to resort to using crutches to get around. Well there it is, I have to sleep on my back for the next six weeks, gout has taken hold, and Nela does her week long soft shoe shuffle up and down the passageway, cooks and washes plates on one leg and makes time to attend me! She is a giant amongst giants! Unfortunately, exhaustion takes its toll!

During all this we have a visit from the Westcourt Community Health nurses on Wednesday who dress my leg wound and will do so for the next six weeks, also help will be forthcoming from the occupational therapists and the dietician!

It is the 26th May 2009, with the week flying past, the pain has subsided somewhat and yet I can just barely shuffle to Gary's car that is parked in our driveway. He will drive me to see Dr Brodie and hopefully, we will be able to put a stop to the inflammation that is causing the problem. Unfortunately, since I am on warfarin for the next six weeks, any inflammation medication cannot be taken because of a possible reaction with both tablets. I grin and bear it!

Back home after seeing the doctor, and Sue has taken Nela shopping as she is now able to walk without crutches. I've decided to watch one of my classic DVD's, "Objective Burma," a 1942 war movie, starring Errol Flynn. Having settled down in my recliner, I watch with interest once more, but doze off, only to awake towards the end of the film. The feet are throbbing but I'm used to it!

About 1.30pm Nela and Sue arrive home from shopping. Nela asks, "Are you hungry and do you want to eat lunch?" I answer in the affirmative and continue watching TV. I must have dozed off for a few minutes because I heard Nela say, "Your lunch is on the table!" I stand and take two steps and promptly turn around and sink back into the recliner.

In a baby like whisper I call Nela. She takes one look at me and said, "What's wrong?" "I don't know, check my blood pressure if it's low, you better call triple zero and get an ambulance here," I croaked. She makes the call and tells the operator that my blood pressure is very low. She is advised to keep me awake and if I need CPR she should administer it to me, "But he has just had a heart operation," she exclaimed. In reply, the operator said, "The CPR takes priority!" Before long a paramedic arrives, who asks, "What's the problem?" "I don't know and I cannot open my eyes, all I can see are colours," I said. Taking my blood pressure that indicated a low 68/53, the paramedic relays the information back to the ambulance service and soon two ambulance units are in the driveway!

Conversations fly around me. Although I try, I still cannot open my eyes. "What's happening, why can't I open my eyes?" I brood, as I'm given oxygen and hear the paramedics say, 'let's get him onto the gurney.' I feel two arms encircle my sternum, and I think 'don't break it!' Then I am lifted and feel that my legs are on an incline, several minutes later I can see, what a relief 'The blood must have gone to my head,' I muse as I am wheeled out of the house to the waiting ambulance. With the oxygen mask covering half my face I notice Darren and Gary looking at me, the latter said, "Everything is alright!" Over the mask I can just see Bella our dog who is enclosed by the swimming pool fence look at me with her saddened eyes.

Travelling in the ambulance for the second time in virtually a week is quite an experience as the unit is fully equipped to handle life threatening situations. The oxygen has helped tremendously. I am now able to take in what is going on around me in what could be a cramped situation. But I am struck once again by the paramedic's efficient and caring manner. I am further impressed by the mentoring that goes on while new paramedics are given extra tutelage in how to do things whilst in a moving vehicle.

I'm feeling much better as we are now in the emergency unit at the Cairns Base Hospital and the inevitable questions are asked, my blood pressure is low at 93/60; blood tests and an x-ray come into play; within a few hours the results indicate that there is a reoccurrence of a low haemoglobin problem. For the second time I am now readmitted into hospital. Further blood transfusions, IV fluids now flow through me, and I am back on the iron tablets. In the course of the week the doctors investigate thoroughly for the cause of the anaemia and to ascertain where and if my blood is leaking somewhere from this now tired body.

Back in Napoleon's days the brave soldiers would have bled to death on ice covered mountains or on war torn battlefields. Fortunately, I've been born in a world of medical technology that is expanding in leaps and bounds.

If my haemaglobin does not reach an acceptable level, then possible invasive investigations such as a colonoscopy or an endoscopy will be the order of the day. However, on 9th July 2009 I did have an endoscopy that showed no evidence of anaemia.

On the 5th day in hospital, I am moved from Med 3 to make room for another patient. I ask the inevitable question, "Where am I going?" The reply was, "You're going to Med 5 it is the penthouse, and it has a much better view of the ocean and the esplanade!" I'm quite happy where I am, although I am not in control of the situation, I say, "Lead on." Med 3, in my opinion was clinically clean and with a fully, energized setting. Wheeled on my bed through the doors of Med 5, I was suddenly engulfed in a wave of depression. I felt as if I was in a sick environment and it did not help matters when I was put next to a non-stop, talkative patient who told me his wife had died in the next ward, two months ago.

Although I call upon my "one point" and try to extend Ki I find that I am unable to breathe in the sickly smell of the ward. My inner energy has somewhat drained away! I find this very unusual, and ask myself, "Why are you feeling this way? Is it because you were moved from friendly surroundings? Has my haemoglobin level reached an all-time low? Is it something sinister that has pervaded my energy lines? Who knows, I cannot explain it!" Nela calls sometime later and knows by the sound of my voice that all is not right. She asks me to tell her what is wrong, but all I can do is mumble a few words. I spend most of my time standing beside the window looking out, and trying to energize myself from the world outside! I finally succeed!

Nela arrives just after lunch on the Sunday just in time to hear the nurse tell me that I would be discharged by 3.00pm. My energy soars as I hear the news. The sense of having your energy sapped and not knowing the cause is a little frustrating. For years I have been doing deep breathing exercises and this was the first time that I felt this way. However, that feeling has disappeared, knowing that in a short time I will be out of hospital, breathing in fresh air. Perhaps it was the culmination of the operation, the gout and the low haemoglobin level that was the trigger? Who knows?

I've returned home and now face the uphill climb of exercising, getting my strength together again to continue my walking program once more! Meanwhile, the community nurses have proceeded to do a wonderful job in dressing my wound; unfortunately, for reasons unknown it had developed a slight infection that is gradually improving.

My weight loss falls from 83kgs to 69kgs and my conversations with the dietician on how to put on weight is proving its worth. Jan has prescribed a multivitamin drink that I enjoy taking each day. Since I had not eaten anything that caused the gout to emerge, she believes, that the weight loss caused a chemical reaction in my body that activated an overload of uric acid to form the tiny crystals that are deposited in the joints causing the joint inflammation, and the ultimate pain. I believe this to be true! It was the only explanation.

I was scheduled for an assessment review by Dr Tam in Townsville on the 18th June 2009, but asked that the appointment be in Cairns the following month, due to my low haemoglobin levels that had seen me hospitalized and all the medical information was in CBH. The cardiac rehabilitation coordinator, Cheryl Hastie was fortunate enough to fit me into Dr Tam's tight schedule for July.

Well, I've fought my own Napoleonic wars and survived. I am glad to say that Nela recovered from her really bad knee sprain and I am on the walking trail once more. Although 35 years of yoga has kept her trim and her mind calm, at this point of time she was very concerned for my health however, she weathered the storm once I was out of trouble. I ponder over the next course that will strengthen my recovery and what lies before me! This period of recovery, was surely the war of attrition for both of us.

Chapter 25
Revitalized!

My operation, eight days of gout, sinus discharge into the throat, rushed to the Cairns Base Hospital twice, courtesy of the Queensland Ambulance Service, into the emergency ward, along the corridors and then into med 3, resulted in a setback. The one week in the Cairns Base Hospital with a low haemoglobin level and several large sachets of blood refills, had taken its toll! After my arrival home I was pussy footing around and trying to do things, however, I was feeling low; and where I had achieved a good walking pace, I was again reduced to a shuffling, hobbling walk!

Little did I know that my phone call to the Cardio Rehab Unit for an appointment, eight weeks after my operation would be the impetus that would put me back on track, for a strong and healthy recovery!

Following directions and entering the third floor lecture room, I was confronted with a table hosting a mini-banquet of assorted nuts, biscuits, a fabulous tasting fruit cake, tea and coffee; I am heartily greeted by a sea of purple people eaters who introduce themselves as Graham, Glen, Tom, Nick, Brian and Anne.

They were former heart patients who had faced their own journey of adversity and recovery; and from their caring demeanor had volunteered their time and services to help other patients work through and successfully achieve their recovery exercise programs. Again, little did I know that their mere presence and their raillery among patients and themselves would lead to the patient's build up of confidence that would improve their recovery time. Been there! Done that! Look at me now, could well be their motto.

A young lass, enters the lecture room and calls my name. She introduces herself to Nela and me as Kylie. Emblazoned on her red shirt and over her left breast was the legend physiotherapist. We walk over to R2D2 where she places a cuff around my left arm, presses the magical button that reveals my blood pressure reading on the monitor screen, the results are then recorded on an exercise form, and then we leave and proceed to the next room

Upon entering, I am engulfed in a time-warp and transported into a jungle military camp complete with camouflage netting, bushes, spiders, snakes and a camp fire hosting a pot of cooking sweets. Then, shaking my head in disbelief, Santa and Mrs. Claus dressed in red, emerge from a smoke, shrouded jungle rainforest, followed by six elves also dressed in red shirts and camouflage shorts, singing Hi! Ho! Hi! Ho! I don't know what you've been told, but Santa's gut has got to go! I must be dreaming! What was in the fruit cake I ate that has given me these hallucinations? I ponder.

Turning my head, I find I am in a field of undulating hills amidst dinosaurs of old, what next? Coming to my senses, I face an array of gymnasium equipment that stand like prehistoric sentinels awaiting the onslaught of humans who will turn them into the joys of active, digital, instruments of fitness. They sound and hum to the tune of, "Take me to your leader, without us you will remain frail and withered; you will remain without a smile, you will not enjoy the laughter! We are your salvation and with your input, your muscles will grow, your heart will pound, your arms and legs will sizzle with a rush of blood, we will help you rid the toxins within your body. You will be alive! Laugh and be happy!"

Kylie interviews me and notes my responses. She then hands me a lap clicker and a timer, then ushers me into the corridor where she tells me that I have to walk from one end of the corridor and back again; with each turn I need to record each full lap and achieve a result in a space of six minutes. I shuffle off and begin with gusto, but soon slow as I become a little tired. This is not me! I should be blitzing this and breaking records, but not today! Finishing off, I find that I have the grand total of 12 laps. "What a wimp! Am I? No way! Stamina is the key to recovery."

However, I must remember that I've just been cut open, operated on and sewn up again, but then each individual is different. We cannot compete against other patients, their exercise program, or against their time level nor their capabilities. I must focus on improving my own physical health. I tell myself that I am not a helpless individual and even if I am slow for the moment, I resolve not to call myself names. Self-pity! 'What is that?' It is not in my vocabulary! *Make no mistake, things will change, on your feet soldier, and move those legs*, I muse as I return the objects of my ordeal to Kylie.

She tells me the program will put me through a series of timed exercises and at the end of each exercise I will be asked the degree of difficulty that ranges from a scale of 0 to 20 on the Borg Scale of Exertion. During these exercises I can talk to her, this will provide a further guide as to how my heart and lung capacity can perform a simple activity that may indicate breathlessness from an out of form, 72 year old, male, physical specimen as me!

Simple as they may seem, I move to the dumbbell weights and start with the lowest weight that has been set for me. I do one set of arm curls that will build up the biceps and then I do a set of the standing shoulder raises that will build up my front shoulders. The axiom is, if it hurts "stop," and advise your purple eater who will take note of it or if it is too painful relay the information to the physio. I am enjoying this exercise because it was exactly what I was doing prior to my operation, but with much heavier dumbbells.

Kylie asks me to sit astride the prehistoric horse and to pull back on the handles of the arm bike. I look at her and sheepishly croak, "Is this okay will it cause problems with my sternum?" In reply she said, "Your sternum is fine, it is strong for this exercise!" I gingerly pull back slowly. Kylie said, "C'mon you can pull faster." Still unsure, I pull slightly faster and detect no pain. Confidence takes over and I begin to pull back in earnest. By the time my alarm rings, I am grinning like a Cheshire cat. I

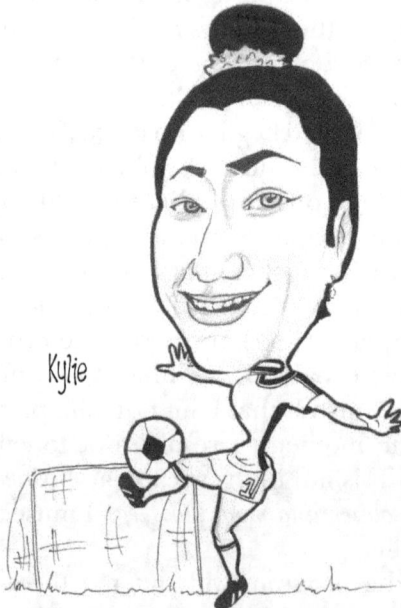

Kylie

can do it! So much for being a pussy cat I thought, as I dismounted off the modern day exercise arm bike.

When I should have been building up my strength I had pussyfooted around at home. I was following the information guide book to recovery concerning carrying and doing things etc. and realized that I had erred too much on the side of caution. Instantly, I knew that the cardio rehab program was not only a confidence builder, but it brought together a group of people with a common interest, a common goal, and that was to improve their well-being.

My two minute step-up exercise begins to take on a rhythm as I step-up, step-down; it is an endless movement where I will never reach the top of the ladder, but I can always reach the bottom. Left, right, up down as I step in place. I'm going no-where, but the knees click and groan, the leg muscle tendons stretch and the heart beats a little faster. No prehistoric animals here! Just the legs and thighs working together to get stronger, ensuring that the heart and lungs reach a beneficial level of capacity through exercise.

The exercise bike stands forlorn, until the stegosaurus within its being, springs to life. I sit and pedal fast, then watch with trepidation as pedal power awakes the digital readout screen that gives me the data of my heart rate, a time clock and the level of resistance that is required to strengthen my legs and thighs. I thank the prophets that I am only on level one as the other levels are harder!

However, as I strap my feet into the footrest of the rowing machine, my mind meanders through the myriad of images that I am sitting on a primeval, cretaceous creature that arises from the depths of the ocean millions of years ago. My rowing machine has a mind of its own, as I am engulfed by a white glow, from a halo of bright, shimmering light that takes me into the past. I slide with bended knees, to straighten once again to the whirring of the pulley and as I pull and bend, I imagine the muscle strength that flows into my legs and shoulders that will eventually affect

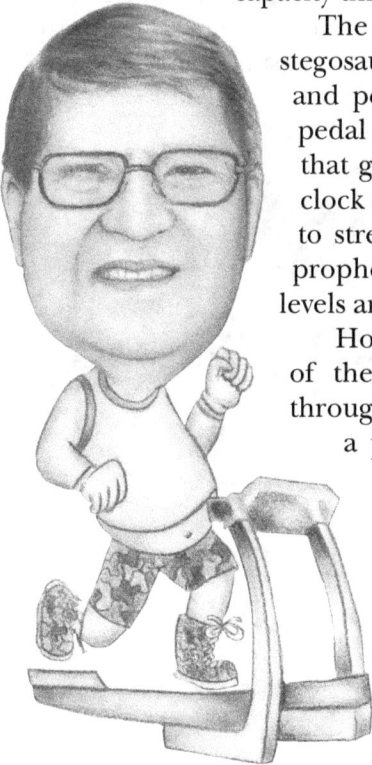

Les

101

a good, muscular, body tone. My heart is beating faster as the seconds roll by and the shoulder muscles take up the strain of each pull. I have reached my two minute limit, the light fades and I take a quantum leap back to reality.

The tension bands are colour-coded, red, yellow, blue, green and black with each having a different resistance value. This exercise strengthens the upper arm biceps and the triceps and the trapezius back muscles; it is also a good indicator if you have a shoulder or sternum pain. You may think it is a waste of time, but if you are going to carry things, then you need to strengthen this area.

The tyrannosaurus rex is dormant until I stand on its body and with a press of a button it starts a slow walk. I am able to increase its speed by pushing another button. For the present I am on 3.0 kpm a normal walking pace I am told for two minutes. Although you can walk the hillside slopes my mission is to walk on the flat ground. The patient beside me is walking 5.0 kpm with a slope of 2 degrees and he seems to be flying. He would if he was on 6.0 kpm! Reaching my time limit, I tell myself that by the end of my program I should be achieving the similar results! Sub-consciously, I add this to my checklist of achievable times.

The exercises have been a symphony of mechanical precision. However, under the baton of Mandi Pashley, our cardiac nurse coordinator; hearts begin to beat faster, as each patient moves his or her hips, legs, or arms to the whirring sounds of a CD that discharges a zumba beat, a rock and roll movement, skipping to the Rocky movie theme, YMCA or to thee upbeat tune of "Mama Mia here we go again," as we bounce on the mini-trampoline or in place throughout the room. The purple eaters have taken up the beat and they extol their mates to do likewise. For me, I have the beat and I'm on the trampoline, my alarm tells me to stop jumping. Back on solid ground and I join the small line, waiting to have their blood

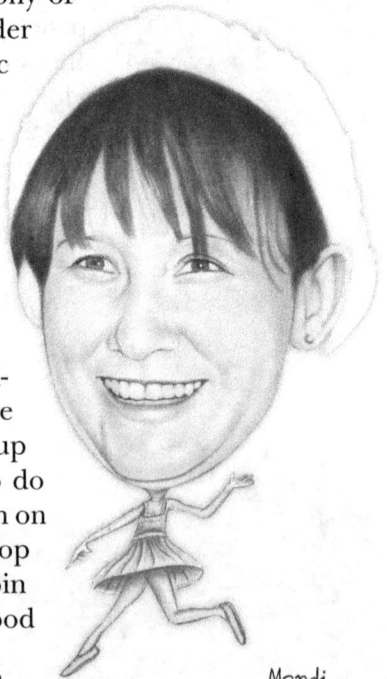

C'mon, let's dance those blues away

Mandi

pressure taken, the cuff is on, the button is pressed and the readout is recorded.

I was introduced to the Wii computer games and what could have been a very sterile environment was transformed into an ambiance of laughter and chuckles. Apart from the games aspect, the patients were unaware of the exercise value that was noteworthy, nor the activities that strengthened the various muscles and the cardio exercises that had the heart pumping. It was something they looked forward to as they really enjoyed doing the Wii program. The use of this program that certainly helped towards the patient's successful recovery because it not only provided the necessary exercises but it enabled them to release their inhibitions. I know I did!

Nevertheless, I cannot stop grinning at the sudden confidence build up within my own mental mind and physical frame. I'm on track and I'm going to make a great recovery. This is my goal and I will enjoy doing it! What an exercise period.

After my cool down exercises, the next stop is the lecture room, for a cup of coffee, biscuits, a slice of cake and a "get to know you," with the other patients. We are waiting for Robert, the psychologist who will speak about "A Different Perspective." Nela and I find the lecture interesting and informative.

Over the next six weeks we will attend a total of 11 lectures with topics ranging from: "You're Heart," "Where to after this?" "Do's and Don'ts," "My Medical List," "From Theory to Practice," "Healthy Eating," "Past, Present and Future," "Increasing Physical Activity," and C.P.R. Each lecture is hosted by experienced people such as a cardiac rehab nurse, health physiotherapist, occupational therapist, a pharmacist, dietician and a general practitioner, this is a well-rounded health information program. In some instances it may bog down during question time, by one or two patients wanting to know the nitty gritty of their own medical problem! Ask questions, by all means, but do not take over the session as going overtime time breaks into the exercise program!

Don't downplay the excellence of the nutritional information. If you really want to lose weight then stick to a plan, it will not happen overnight but it will happen! Following the dieticians advice I am still maintaining my weight between 76 to 77.5 kgs and I'm feeling a lot better for it, this is after I dropped from 83kg to 69 kgs during my hospitalization.

It's Thursday, Nela and I are having our coffee and listening to the chatter of other patients. Max, my buddy from Townsville is sitting beside me, when like a zephyr over a clear blue sea, the bubbling, effervescent

Mandi in her red shirt promenades across the floor doing her chasse. Within seconds laughter bounces off the walls and ceiling as the banter begins in earnest from the purple eaters, the patients, who are chuckling with laughter over the anecdotes or tales from the ever-smiling Mandi. Keeping it alive is surely our motto for laughter!

Unfortunately, the red shirts that added a glow to our cardiac nurses and the physiotherapists have been withdrawn by the bureaucracy for something that is dull and ever so close to those worn by the customer service officer in a supermarket! The heart is red, the blood is red, so bring back the red shirts as they are recognizable and more importantly it epitomizes the work the cardiac staff do with heart patients.

Prior to the commencement of the exercise program, the count down to zero, fast approaches, and under the direction of our exercise guru Graham, we enter into an activity spin that will warm up our muscles. Commencing with shoulder rotations, neck and shoulder stretches, arm stretches, knee raises on the spot and his coup de grace where the right elbow touches the left knee raise and vice versa. John, a patient, was going exceptionally well, except he was bringing his knee straight up rather than across on the diagonal. Laughter within the group was poetry in motion!

When Mandi is unavailable, Anita Basu or Kylie takes over, but in this case Kylie is replaced by Kylie Sommerville, the cardio rehab physiotherapist who has been away on maternity leave. Kylie prepares and plans each individual exercise program and flits from patient to patient making sure that they are achieving their own personal goals and doing the exercises correctly.

Since my foray into my first exercise program last Tuesday, I now look forward to the physical exercises during the weeks ahead, but alas! It is time for another setback! Awaking on Sunday I head off to the airport to collect our relations from Canada and feel a slight twinge behind my left ankle but take no notice! However, Monday morning is a different story. I had been forewarned by yesterday's twinge and suddenly find I can hardly walk. It can't be gout! 'Now what have I done?' I ponder getting into my car and driving off to see the doctor!

My G.P. has called for an x-ray that has indicated that I have an inflamed Achilles tendon, rest and ice is the order of the day, resulting in having to cancel next Thursday's rehab. I am not in the least amused, I can no longer go for my usual 30 minute walks without feeling the pain, and it certainly has interfered with my recovery time. Fortunately, I have the dumbbells to keep myself busy, the bike and the swimming pool to

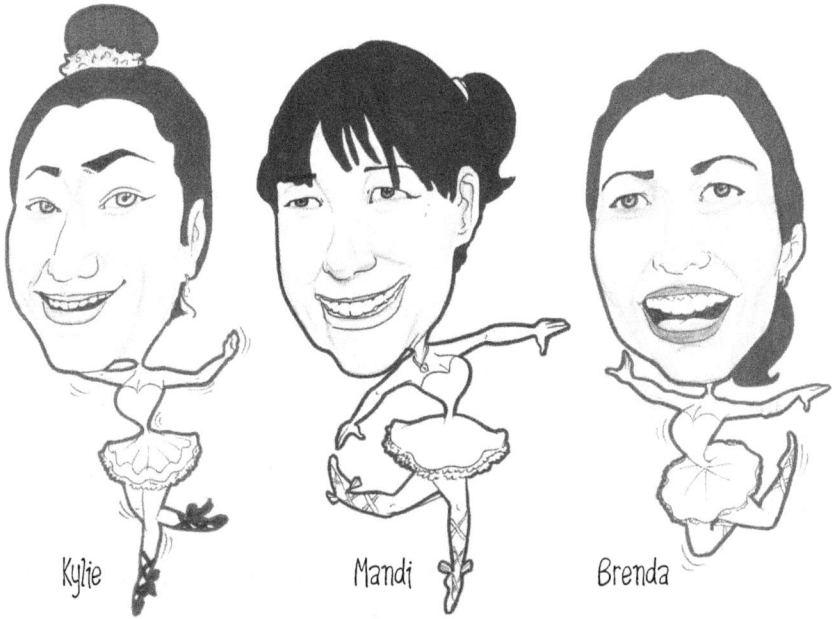

Kylie   Mandi   Brenda

Laughter is from the heart

exercise the legs and arms; icing every hour and slow stretches of the tendon has been helpful. I don't believe this has occurred, what next as my mind lingers over the question?

Why all these setbacks to prevent me from walking? It seems the gods are fearful that I will crack the bitumen road foundations or is it that I may trip and fall and damage the road surface of my face and arms! Whatever the frustration, I ensure that my stretches are done correctly and not overdone, and that I will be fit for the following week of rehab.

The six week exercise program flies past and before I know it Mandi and Kylie have presented me with my certificate of participation. I tell them that they will not get rid of me so quickly and enquire whether a vacancy exists for another purple eater like myself.

Mandi and Kylie believe there is room for one more and they tell me to make an appointment to see Anne Chirio, the FNQ Hospital Foundation volunteer coordinator. Weeks later I receive a phone call from Anne asking me to come in and collect my purple shirt and identification tags. Wow! I am elated as this gives my life an extra lift, because I will find myself caught up in the infection of singing, dancing and indulging in repartee with my fellow volunteers, the patients, Mandi and Kylie. Revitalize, go with the flow and enjoy the exercise program of Santa's cardio rehab boot camp. *This is not the end but the beginning,* I reflect replacing the telephone on its stand.

Upon reflection, the program was of considerable help towards my recovery. The banter with the old and new patients was stimulating and significant, because it opened up their fear of the unknown in relation to soreness, pain and their post op experiences; they had the opportunity to compare their own problems with people who had similar heart difficulties. The main aim was to build confidence and to motivate oneself into achieving good results.

My first months as a purple eater, is more than uplifting, it's put pep into my step! I gaze upon the faces of our new patients who have entered the jungle rehab boot camp. They wonder with some trepidation as to what they are going to do! Nevertheless, their fears are allayed when they come face to face with their first purple eater, who takes them through their exercise regimen, offering explanations as to how the exercise will benefit them. They ask questions and are inquisitive as to what type of operations that we ourselves had gone through, to where we are today?

During the course of their exercise program they must think the purple eaters are a "crazy, zany bunch of volunteers," but if it brings a smile or laughter to their faces, then, we have achieved a major goal towards helping their recovery.

However, there are a few who have entered the program without having exercised in a gym or used the prehistoric creatures of equipment that are all alien to them, but are eagerly awaiting their pleasure. Then there are those who have already programmed their own minds, that the exercise program is a complete waste of their time. They do it once and fail to continue the rehab program.

We try to dispel this myth and through our own experiences we try to show them the value of doing the physical exercise program correctly. Of course, we have those who believe that they can go through the exercises at speed and on full throttle, and nothing will deter them in slowing down to get the full benefit from the activities. They may question why they can only lift light weights, "I'm strong enough to lift the heavier ones," they acclaim! They forget that the nature of their body has been interfered with, the chest has been cut open and the miracle of the medical surgeons have poked, prodded parts of the body that are not used to the human touch.

The purple eaters encourage positive vibes. Hopefully, we build up the confidence of the patient; we try to make them feel good about themselves and what they are achieving through the exercise program. We talk about their goals for the future and we instil, we hope, a sense of focus for their well-being.

Not-withstanding, there are the courageous, and none more worthy than Bob, a diabetic for some years, has heart and plumbing repairs etc. He is happy, boisterous and gives more cheek than all the purple eaters together. We love him! He puts more effort into the exercises than any one patient; he sweats as if he is in a sauna; but above all, is his attitude, that all is not lost. He loves to joke and tells quite a few, whether he is pedaling flat out on the treadmill or doing his step-ups; he plays at Cinderella when we place the ankle weight around his good, right leg and the other around the steel shaft of his prosthesis! You guessed it he has lost a leg below the knee.

I was telling him about a guy from overseas who had been given a bionic hand. He said, "I'd give my left leg for a bionic one and I'll paint it black." Mystified, I said, "Why paint it black?" "When I'm walking in the dark, you won't be able to see it," bursting out with laughter as he continued raising his leg weights. He had all of us chuckling! Attitude! He has more attitude than I'll ever have, but he is a hero who faces adversity with laughter; he wants to live life to the fullest. Robert we salute you! "Dum Vivimus, Vivamus!" (While we live, let us live!)

Nevertheless, there are others who provide inspiration as they exercise and battle the pain that is causing havoc emotionally to their bodies, or those that have fallen to another adversity other than their heart problems. The purple eaters become quite aware of some of the emotional problems and through our gentle demeanor and caring we hope that our frivolity and our conversations might lessen some of the emotional strains they face.

December 2nd 2009, and Santa and Mrs. Claus have re-emerged from their jungle retreat and entered the safety haven of Santa's cardio rehab boot camp where there is much laughter as the jovial competition judges enter the hospital retreat to cast their votes for the best Ward display. We've provided a song, stories, a camp fire and a well-displayed jungle environment but at the end of the day we find that we have come second. This has not deterred us as we have put our combined creative minds for a better display and genre in 2010. Being in the pink, the rehab, lights up our hearts and performs the miracle of rebuilding wasted muscle tissue back to their former glory.

Our pre-Christmas lunch for our small group and the bigger Christmas party for all our former and newer patients was a highlight for

2009 as new and old got together to converse about how well they have recovered and what they are doing with their life.

The year 2010 and the months have marched on, and last September 28 the FNQ Hospital Foundation provided a breakfast for all the volunteers and awarded certificates of service. I was pleasantly surprised when my name was called out, and handed my certificate of having reached my one year of service. The months had not marched they flew like the speed of light through the universe. My purple eater colleagues had amassed a total of some 32 years between them, whilst two female volunteers accepted their awards for 20 years of service each; what an outstanding achievement! "Way to go," I quietly exclaimed, as I sipped my cup of coffee.

Meanwhile, the cardio rehab program carries on, Mandi and Kylie interview new patients; the warm-ups are completed and the new patients are taken under our wings, except for the patients who are mid way through the program and know what to do, but the purple eaters remain vigilant and watch them perform their exercises correctly. Mandi has moved to the Tuesday sessions and Yvonne has entered the scene on the Thursday to carry out her duties of holding hands with R2D2 and pressing the all important button that sets the machine blinking with delight, and the figures jostle each other to produce the blood pressure reading.

The first group is finished by 10am and after their last blood pressure reading, the patients retire to the lecture room to await the visiting speaker. They comfortably relax with their cup of tea or coffee, partake of a slice of Ann's famous fruit cake or nibble on a couple of biscuits.

Meanwhile, administration officer Bill O'Reilly-Smith continues to make his unassuming presence felt as he checks records and completes his paperwork by appearing and disappearing like a phantom floating between the trees surrounding the boot camp.

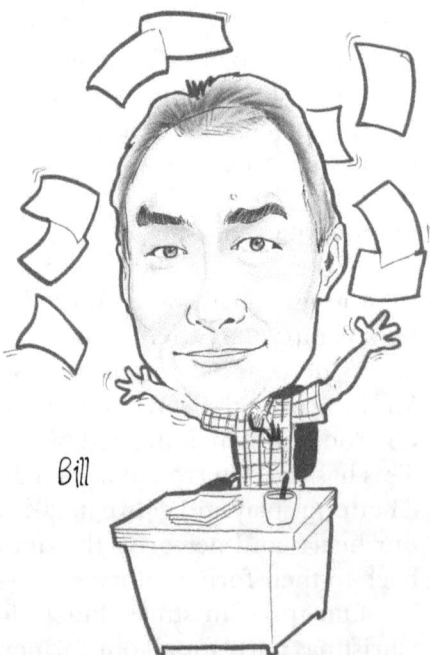

Bill

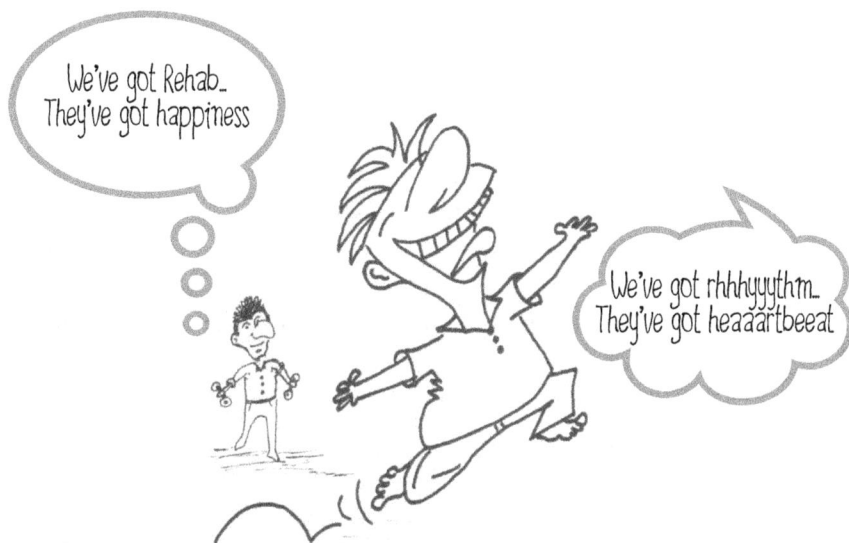

Happiness is completing the six week Educational and Physical Cardiac Rehab Program. The major contributor to a person's physical motivation is working with a group of people having similar problems. We watch with delight as much older patients give their all to regain fitness. Some patients travelled up to 350 kms to participate in this group therapy. The program instills confidence in one's ability to change to a new lifestyle. Happiness is continuing on and maintaining your fitness level. You were faced with a wonderful group of Cardiac Nurses, Physiotherapists and a zany bunch of delightful volunteers who provided you with extra motivation.

In the meantime, the purple people eaters have moved down to the staff canteen. We make our coffee and sit around a rectangular and somewhat wobbly table. We munch on our sandwiches and sip our coffee or tea as we solve the problems of the nation, the government and the leaders and the rising costs that hit the pockets of the ordinary citizen. We discuss our own life experiences and marvel what we have achieved in our life time. We visit memory lane and retell anecdotes of the past and the present, often erupting in laughter, this fortifies us for the second exercise session.

Graham relates his air force accomplishments and several experiences in Manila as Tom sprinkles three satchets of salt over his beloved curry and rice and reminisces of his hottest curry with a group of army Gurkhas during his war exploits. Glen is our I.T. man he provided us with up to date computer information and where to travel in this vast country of ours. Anne had hid the salt shaker from Tom but he soon discovered it, she is our famous fruit cake maker. Meanwhile Nick the 'Benny Hill' of our little troupe settles down to organizing his cup of tea and sandwiches onto his serviette. Brian and I recollect our time in P.N.G. Brian was an army engineer stationed in Port Moresby, who coached of a rugby team from Marshall Lagoon. Ironically I spent five years teaching at the Kelerakwa Primary school in the same area.

Working in the Cardio Rehab Unit has been most gratifying, especially working side by side with such fine, dedicated and caring people. To be able to play a small part in helping other heart patients achieve their own recovery program successfully has been enlightening, enjoyable and rewarding.

My journey as a volunteer is just beginning! Yet I have come through

Cardiac Rehab Volunteers

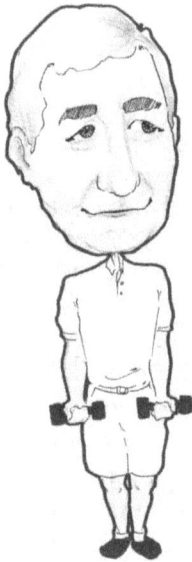

Nick

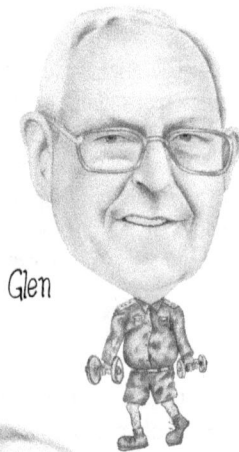

Glen

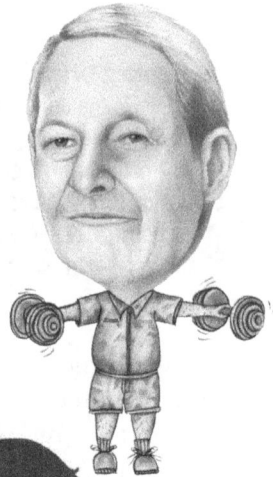

Brian

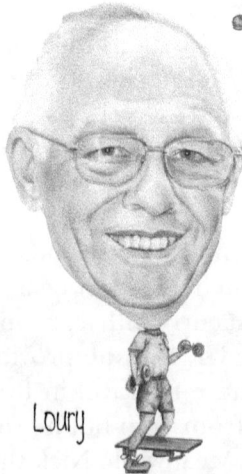

Loury

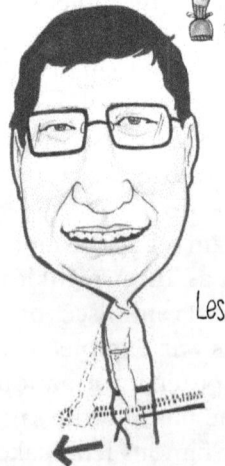

Les

a full 360 degree circle from the time I had to cancel our vacation in February 2009 to once again fulfilling our Philippine dream trip.

There is a strong rumour that the Cardiac Rehabilitation Unit will be moved from the Cairns Base Hospital to the Cairns North Community Health Centre in the New Year. If this occurs I will be saddened as one of my goals was to have at least 15 years volunteer service with the FNQ Hospital Foundation.

Well! It Happened! The Unit did move to the Community Health Centre into a room and in my opinion that was inadequate in size to cater for the number of patients, volunteers and visiting student physiotherapists. Exercising in a cramped gym will lead to patients having unnecessary injuries. Heaven forbid.

Volunteers became furniture removalists as we moved chairs and tables to cater for the patients before and after their exercise program. We did not have a permanent lecture room as previously at the hospital. What was missing was the all important bed for a patient who became unwell or faced a waiting game for an ambulance to take him/her to hospital. I believe a wheelchair or a folding bed would be beneficial as we do not want heart patients being under more stress than necessary. Initially we continually tripped over the protruding back leg of the chairs but to offset this problem the powers to be put red tape around the back legs, of course who looks downwards! Nevertheless as volunteers we coped and ensured that patients were successful in completing their own exercise programs safely.

Cardiac Rehab Volunteers

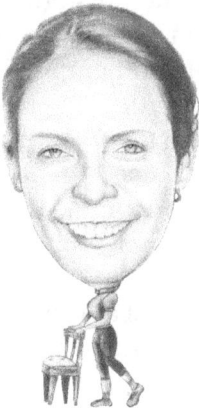 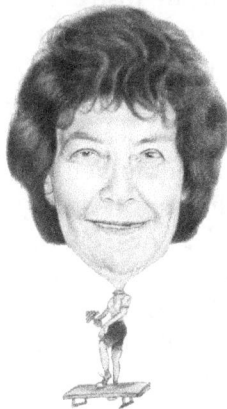 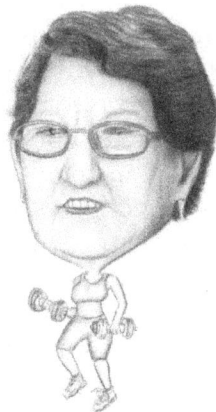

Karen   Ann   Anne

Chapter 26
The Cardiac Rehab Volunteer

My fellow volunteers and I have something in common. Between us we probably had a coronary bypass artery graft (CABG), an aortic valve replacement, a pacemaker or stents inserted into our elderly torsos.

By nature we have an amiable manner and a pleasing disposition. I believe we have very good communication and people skills that are necessary in fostering and building confidence within the patients. We believe that we can instill the confidence for them to continue building their strength towards their new healthy life style after accomplishing their rehabilitation program. We often relate our own operation experiences that further helps towards motivating the patient into gaining their confidence and bettering their own exercise performance. We are ever mindful of patient information confidentiality.

It is our attitude towards good teamwork that provides a healthy environment within the relationship between patient, fellow volunteers, the physiotherapist and the cardiac rehabilitation clinical nurse and staff.

We are concerned with the patient's welfare with a strong sense of responsibility as we carry out the instructions set by the physiotherapist during the patients six week rehabilitation exercise program. We ensure that we advise the cardiac clinical nurse or the physiotherapist if the patient shows some distress or muscle weakness during their exercises.

We are mindful of the various age differences and aware of the risks generally in their use of the equipment. Nevertheless, as the patient's confidence grows and their exercise program nears its end, they are permitted to safely manage their own exercises with minimal supervision. The volunteers are aware of the situation and constantly "watchful" over the patient's movements during the exercise period. Still I am concerned that it takes only a nano second for a situation to occur and who takes responsibility for this occurrence?

On completion of each patient's blood pressure reading we commence the rehabilitation exercises with several Warm- ups:

- **Marching on the spot** - will help increase the heart rate flow and pump the blood through our plumbing system into the entire body.

- **Shoulder rotations** - warm up the neck and shoulder support muscles until we feel a mild stretch. Continue marching.

- **Arm rotations** - post surgical patients should be careful. Perform this exercise gently. This warms up the shoulder rotator cuff and stretches out the thoracic spine. Rotations should not rise above the 90 degrees.

- **Abductors and adductors** - These are the primary support muscles for the hips. Legs spread apart (double the width of the shoulders) side lunge left side, feel the muscle stretch. Hold for an eight count then side lunge to the right side. Correct stretching technique is required as these muscles are used in lower limb activities.

- **Mini squats** - feet shoulder width apart, toes pointing ahead, warm-up the quads, hamstring and gluteal muscles, knee bends should be small and comfortable for the patient. These muscles will be used in the step-up and sit to stand (squat) exercises.

- **Ankle rotations** - hold on to something to maintain stability and balance, feet close to the ground, rotate ankle gradually increasing in size.

- **Marching on the spot** - This relaxes the body and has minimized tension as the muscles that have been stretched return to a comfortable position with the added bonus of increasing the heart rate and circulation to the larger muscle groups.

Each new patient receives his or her exercise program and is coupled

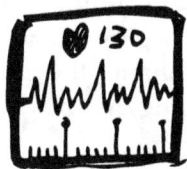

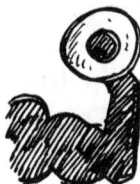

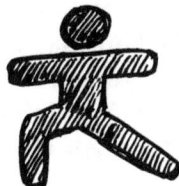

with a volunteer while others may commence with minimal supervision but are under the watchful eyes of the volunteers. The patient records the degree of difficulty after each exercise. Our Rehabilitation exercises are as follows:

- **Dumbbell weights – bicep curls/shoulder raises/lateral raises**
- **Wall Push-ups**
- **High or low step-ups**
- **Resistance (tension) Bands**
- **Sit to Stand (squats)**
- **Treadmill**
- **Ankle weights (calf raises, side raise & back raise)**
- **Fixed bike**
- **Cross-Country trainer**
- **Rowing machine – push with legs/pull/keep back straight/ release/arm/legs**
- **Further Blood Pressure reading**

Cool down stretches include shoulder stretches, standing calf stretch, hamstring stretch and quadriceps stretch.

Morning tea and a one hour informative education lecture completes the Tuesday and Thursday morning cardiac rehabilitation program that lasts for six weeks.

To put it into better perspective I have produced a "Swim Lane Diagram" (Rummler- Brache Diagrams) the flow chart will help the patient understand the integrating process between the Cardiac Clinical Nurse Coordinator, the physiotherapist and the volunteer and how the process leads to their physical improvement during their the six week rehabilitation program.

I believe the swim lane diagram to be better suited in describing the above integrating process rather than a flow chart that shows the chief at the top with the other personal falling into areas of responsibility. More-so when trying to label volunteers as public servants in the broad sense. The swim lane diagram provides that the patient begins with and finishes with the Cardiac Clinical Nurse Coordinator. At a glance the patient has a general picture of what to expect when under-going the six week cardiac rehabilitation program.

Steps to Rehab

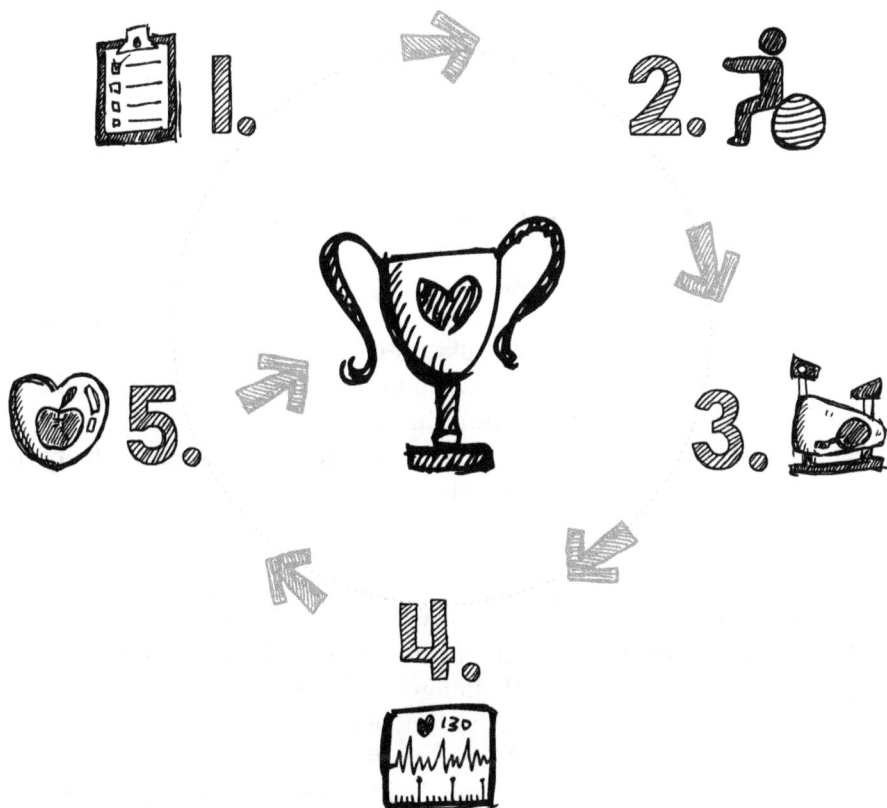

1. Cardiac Clinical Nurse Coordinator	• Patient interview – discuss Rehab Program • Blood Pressure (BP) readings • Current health issues before commencing Rehab Program
2. Physiotherapist	• Patient interview – discuss exercise • Test patient • Introduce new patient to Cardiac Rehab Volunteers

3. Volunteers *Explain, demonstrate and monitor exercises*	GROUP AND INDIVIDUAL SESSIONS COMMENCE • Volunteer explains exercises • Group warm up exercises – new patient with Volunteer mentor • Volunteer stresses importance of exercising slow and with good technique • Records degree of perceived exertion after each timed or set exercise – mid and final • BP reading – Cool down exercises • Records how patients feel and their progress
4. Physiotherapist	• Discuss exercise program with patient – stress the importance of the perceived exertion rating • Discusses any health issues arising from the exercise Program • Checks final BP • Writes up new exercise sets
5. Cardiac Clinical Nurse Coordinator	AFTER 6 WEEKS • Patient interview – discuss health issues, challenges with new lifestyle after operation, and Rehab • Patient graduates from Rehab Program • Hospital will follow-up with a phone call

Informative Educational Health lectures with visiting speakers are part of the program

Quite often new patients are overwhelmed when they come to the Unit and find that there are other patients waiting for the exercises to begin. They may have a sense of "What am I here for...? I've never been to a gym before! What do they expect me to do? I'm too weak to attempt all those 'exercises. Then there is the younger patient who enters the Rehab Unit to be confronted with much older people, what are their thoughts? Do they feel depressed? Rest assured the Cardiac Rehabilitation Unit is there to ensure that you take your time, build up muscle tone and confidence in yourself to be able to tackle the work you will face at home and at your place of work. Believe in the program and when you complete it you will want to carry on.

I would like to point out the importance of the **Borg Rating of Perceived Exertion Scale** that is based on how a patient perceives the physical sensations he feels during his physical activity. This includes an increase in his heart rate, muscle fatigue, increased sweating or out of breath. By providing an honest rating of difficulty the physiotherapist is able to adjust the rate of intensity of the set exercises as to how hard the patient's body is working, by increasing or decreasing the exercise load. The perceived exertion rating then provides the patient with a self-monitoring scale that reflects his own feelings during heavy and active work at home.

"Huff! Puff! Huff! Puff!" A rating of "**17** – "Very hard" it is very strenuous. The feeling may be very heavy or being very tired.

"Pheeew!" The scale of "**13** – "Somewhat hard" the patient perceives it was hard but it was OK to continue.

Oh! "It was a walk in the park!" This was a "**9** – "Very light" The patient is able to continue without exerting himself.

During the exercises the volunteers monitor the patient through the Talk Test that provides an indication to his level of effort. For instance, if you can talk but not sing your rating could be classified as a moderate intensity activity. On the other hand not being able to say more than a few words without pausing for breath would indicate that you are doing a vigorous intensity activity. Since I don't feel like talking to myself I use my **whistling** test in rating my exertion when at home.

We are a zany bunch of volunteers and at time we may be boisterous because of the laughter we generate that certainly uplifts a patient's spirit after their major operation. Perhaps others resent the noise factor, but then, why shouldn't we rejoice that we are alive knowing that the best medicine is laughter and we do not dwell on self pity or being miserable. Appreciate life, laugh and be happy.

We congratulate and welcome Karen, Les, Bill, Michael and James into our ranks as we are a dedicated group of volunteers who take pride in helping new patients regain their confidence after their initial cardiac operation. I believe that this confidence stems from the fact that all the volunteers have undergone similar operations. We are the purple people eaters and we are family.

It would be remiss of me if I did not mention our relieving cardiac nurses Jaquie, Anita, Karen, Natalia, Lee, Tania and Trudie together with our physiotherapists Kelli, Tony, Trent and Sophie who have graced our

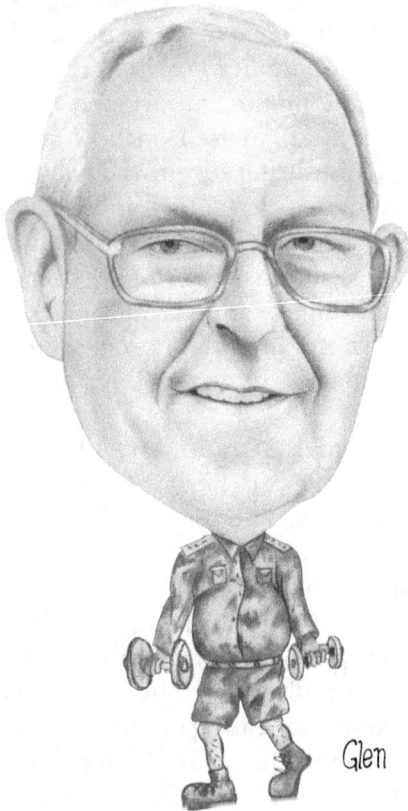

Glen

portals with their experience to work with our cardiac patients. What a wonderful group of people to work with and to gain knowledge from their wealth of experiences.

April-May 2015, we are saddened by the loss of our two old stalwarts Tom and Glen who passed away within weeks of each other; they will be sadly missed. Glen was the mainstay behind our cardiac nurses and the volunteers. Time was nothing to him as he would arrive well before 7: 00a.m. to set up the projector, seating and organizing the necessary paperwork. Outside the Rehab Unit he was busy at his beloved bowls club and coaching the many who wanted to play Bowls, together with his committee commitments. He would take us on a memory journey and his love for fishing to the amazing beachside of Merimbula located on the southern New South Wales coast.

To enlarge our family of patients, x-patients and those who become our new rehab patients, rejoice! Happy Hearts will start up again, so keep in touch.

Chapter 27
Ki Development

People often say relax, but how do you relax? Do you let your muscles slump? Do you know that when you relax correctly you are strong? Have an open mind and learn about your Ki development.

Ki is universal energy, capable of infinite expansion and contraction, which can be directed, but not contained by the mind. The basic principles of Ki are a way of bringing light to one's natural strength and hidden abilities by letting your energy flow. The goal of Ki training is mind and body coordination in any activity, including sleep. It is relatively easy to unify, mind and body while standing or sitting, but much more difficult to maintain in movement. In developing Ki, students study relaxation exercises, breathing methods, meditation and Kiatsu Therapy. (Book of Ki: Co-ordinating Mind and Body in Daily Life by Koichi Tohei-1976)

The Four Basic Principles

1. Keep One Point
2. Relax completely
3. Keep Weight Underside
4. Extend Ki

The following exercises are simple and if done daily will become an automatic response and will help you to alleviate your tendency to stress. **I dare you to try it for a month!** Keep an open mind. Learn your mantra. Make it an automatic thought each time you do something.

You are strong when you relax through Ki development

KI BREATHING EXERCISE 1

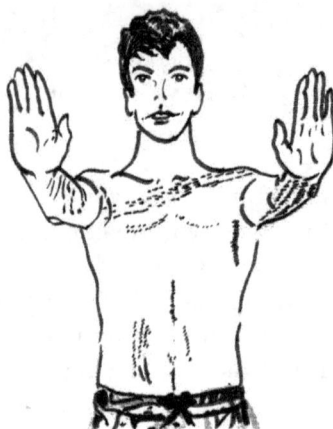

Stand with your feet about shoulder width apart. Breathe in gently through your nose. Raise your hands, palms forward in front of your shoulders. Exhale slowly through your mouth, using the **'Haa'** sound, as you do so, push your hands straight forward until your arms are fully extended in front of you.

Breathe in again and slowly allow your hands to return in front of your shoulders.

For variety, as you exhale push your hands to either side or straight above you or downwards to your waist, or combine the four movements each time you breathe in through your nose and exhale through your mouth.

For example:

- Inhale from your **ONE POINT** to your shoulders
- Exhale and extend your hands in front of you
- Inhale and return your hands to your shoulders
- Exhale and push your hands straight above your head
- Inhale slowly and return your hands to your **ONE POINT**

You are strong when you relax through Ki development

KI BREATHING EXERCISE 2

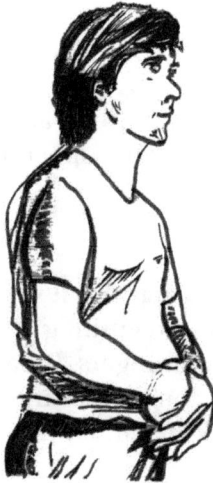

When you complete your breathing exercises, cross your hands over your **ONE POINT**. Close your eyes, gently inhale through your nose and visualise the air flowing through to your **ONE POINT** and *extend your Ki* by slowly exhaling.

Concentrate on your breathing, think **ONE POINT** and *extend Ki each time you exhale*. After a few minutes, go into normal breathing and as you exhale, think of your **ONE POINT** getting smaller and smaller, and as you inhale it becomes bigger.

Now I want you to try and think of nothing but your breathing. You have your hands over your **ONE POINT**, your knees will slightly sag; you may begin to sway slightly or even faster. Let it happen, go with it, you will not fall over. Try to extend your exercise time from five minutes to longer.

If you cannot focus because of background noise, say, "I acknowledge all noise; as it enters my right ear it will filter out to nothing through my left ear".

How to...

Get Your "ONE POINT" "Breathe In"

- Take a small, sniff of air, as if you are smelling a flower
- Visualize the air flowing down from your nose, throat, shoulders, chest stomach, to your ONE POINT which is located two inches below your navel.
- • Think "One Point," the air sinks down and your stomach protrudes. Feel the weight come off your shoulders

"Extend Ki" "Breathe Out"

- **Extend Ki by visualizing the flow** through the stomach, chest, shoulders, and arm and gushing along your relaxed arm and out through your relaxed fingers. Breathe out, **using an ahh sound!** The stomach now compresses into your body. Use a final 'uff' sound to exhale all the air, hold for three seconds then breathe in.

- **You can extend this Ki to any part of your body**, visualize the painful area and focus by extending your Ki to it. Then breathe out all the poisonous toxins from your body or breathing out all the negative thoughts that you have in your mind.

- **Take several sniffs of air in and visualize it going to your ONE POINT**, now extend Ki by breathing slowly out of your mouth making an 'AHHH' sound. **Do this at least 10 times**. You can do this quietly to yourself when walking, sitting in your car at the stop lights, driving or sitting in an Office, on a bus etc. Feel the weight coming off your shoulders. **Mantra – Get "ONE POINT and Extend Ki."**

- **When you wake up in the morning**, sit on the side of the bed; place your hands lightly on your thighs.

- **Breathe in – get your one point** – if you are being distracted by noise – acknowledge it – say, 'I acknowledge all types of noise – the noise enters my right ear and filters out through my left –"I am now focused."

- how do you feel?

- **You are ready for the day's work.**

Now that you have learnt this, you can start to visualize your ONE POINT getting smaller from the size of the moon to a microdot flying through the Universe as you breathe out.

- When you inhale think of that microdot getting bigger, and bigger as a full moon. (ten times) Try thinking of 'nothing.' Focus!
- **Get your ONE POINT and EXTEND YOUR Ki** throughout the day will give you that extra energy. When you are sitting for exams, walking, picking up something from the floor, carrying a heavy item, gardening, digging, etc **just say the Mantra, "Get One Point and Extend Ki"**
- **Make this an automatic thought.** This is my daily mantra! Make it yours!
- You can do it!

Remember:

- **When you are standing - weight is underside.**
- **When sitting – weight is underside**
- **When lying down on your back – weight is underside**

Exercise 1 (Standing)

- Breathe in – get your one point
- Breathe out – extend Ki
- Do this 10 times
- Stand with your hands across your one point
- Focus on 'nothing' – you knees will slightly sag as you think of your one point - you may find yourself beginning to sway slowly – don't fight it – let it happen – it may even become a faster — relax – don't tighten up. You will not fall.
- When the swaying stops stay in the standing position – do not straighten your knees- after 10 minutes of trying to think of "nothing" finish off – clap your hands and rub the energy into your face and over your body. How do you feel?

Exercise 2

- You need a friend
- Extend your arm, to about a 60 degree angle, clench your fist and tense it.
- Your friend now uses both his hands to bend the arm back towards your shoulder. Note the pressure used. Note the tension you used.
- Now do the same thing except unclench your fist and relax the hand. Bend your elbow to about 60 degrees, extending your hand and fingers outward. Get your 'one point', then extend your Ki by visualizing water gushing through your arm and out through your fingers like a fire hose.
- Your friend now tries to bend your arm back to your shoulder. Note the pressure.
- You can talk to your friend during this part of the exercise.
- You can now see the difference between 'tense' pressure and that relaxed position of extending your Ki, which was stronger?

Exercise 3

- Lying on your back
- Get Your One Point
- Think weight underside (don't fight it!)
- Feel the weight coming off your shoulders, feel your head bending back slightly, visualize the weight falling from all parts of your body
- You can stay in this relaxed position from 10 -30 minutes
- Try this before sleeping and you will fall asleep naturally.
- If you are unable to lie on your back then sit on a chair upright, but do not use the back rest. Continue with the exercise.
- I do this while I am sitting in the car waiting for the lights to change. Just the thought will get you to your 'one point.

My Favourite Exercise

- In a standing position, raise right leg and place the foot on the opposite left knee.
- Get ONE POINT, think of an unmovable rock that cannot fall over.
- Extend your right arm, but not locked, have somebody push your thumb on the extended arm to push you backward and off balance. Think ONE POINT
- Great fun! When they realize that they cannot move you off balance except for your natural arm movement.

Think ONE POINT and EXTEND Ki in everything you do, make it an automatic thought i.e. sitting, walking, picking up something etc. You will find that you have energy, you will not flinch with a sudden noise, and you will have achieved inner calmness. Keep it up! Try it for thirty days! Has it helped you? Enjoy the experience! If you're angry! Get your 'one point' and extend Ki that will bring about an inner calmness within your mind and body.

Remember not to become a VCR and think negative thoughts that make you sick. Do not continually tell your body that you are sick because your sub -conscious mind acts on your instructions

Chapter 28
Guiding Hands

Lighting the Way. The following quote by Mother Teresa entitled, 'On Kindness' epitomizes the nature of a person's character towards others.(search quotes.com)

"Spread love everywhere you go. First of all in your own house...
let no one ever come
To you without leaving better and happier,

Be the living expression of God's kindness;
Kindness in your face, kindness in your eyes,
Kindness in your smile and kindness in your warm greeting."

There comes a time when you must rely on the friendship, love, caring and kindness from persons close to you. People do make a difference in your life; they give hope, encouragement and generosity in their deeds because in some way you are special to them.

Falling into this area of excellence are our neighbours of 22 years Sue and Gary Schofield; Marietta (Mayet) Percali and her daughter Sharleen, who between them gave us that helping hand when it was needed. Both families gave of their time to take Nela shopping; to take me to my doctor's appointments or to drive us to the Cairns Base Hospital for me to attend my cardio rehab exercise program. In most cases they waited around until I had finished or drove back to pick us up a later time. Sometimes we took the scenic bus route around the city and the Esplanade to the Lake Street bus terminal where we switched from one bus to another that ferried us to the Stockland, Earlville shopping centre.

It is difficult to find the right words of praise and appreciation, but we are indebted to them for their acts of kindness and caring, more-so for the words of encouragement that uplifted me towards a successful recovery.

They were concerned when they first saw me on my arrival home from the Townsville hospital. They knew me as a physically fit young man of 72 but had to face a skinny specimen who had lost 14 kgs over the hospitalization period. I learnt later, that they were visibly shaken during my second ambulance pick up with half my face covered by the oxygen mask! For a split second the seed of 'what if... occurred, Played on their minds?' Their friendship has and always will provide a stimulus of enrichment that has impacted on both Nela and I, leaving a lasting impression.

Our first incursion into shopping by ourselves was an ordeal, customers and sightseer's scurried from one place to another, bustling as if on an important mission of buy! Buy! Meanwhile I was leaning and propelling our trolley through a maddening crowd at a pace that even a tortoise could beat me; the trolley was my winning post and if it had been a hurdles race, it was all over red rover for me! I would have been flat on my face without its guiding support!

On the contrary, the Far North Queensland ambulance service and their select army of paramedics are without doubt a fine group of dedicated men and women. They deserve all the credit that can be bestowed upon them. Their friendly manner, calm demeanor, caring attitude and their professionalism that they displayed in transporting me on two different occasions to the Cairns Base Hospital emergency unit was outstanding. I was further impressed by their efficient ability to insert a cannula into my arm whilst in a moving vehicle and to mentor the newer paramedics while on the move was exemplary.

They deserve our continual support and the government assistance to ensure they are able to provide personnel development for their team members and to upgrade equipment and machines that helps them in their professional capacity to care for and the movement of the patients to hospital.

Likewise, to all the doctors, nurses and support staff that performed their own specific miracles of helping towards my recovery was more than fantastic. Equally important were the personnel who manned the emergency unit, not only did they do their best but at times endure the wrath of frustrated patients with a caring calmness and a smile.

Conversely, I must thank Tony Franz, General Manager and Anne Chirio Volunteer Coordinator of the Far North Queensland Hospital Foundation for giving me the opportunity of becoming a volunteer with the people purple eaters. The 320 registered purple shirt volunteers, who unselfishly give of their time to help others is outstanding, especially when you total up their years of service to the Foundation. They host a yearly breakfast and Christmas lunch for the volunteers with the distribution of certificates of appreciation for years of service. The foundation through sponsorship and fundraising events provides grants and purchases vital medical equipment, to help research and education, to support health care provisions in Far North Queensland.

The old car park now stands forlorn and awaits its demolishment, for a new hospital wing to be built, whilst across the road a new edifice hosts the Foundation's new offices and the new car park has its share of teething problems. None more than a frustrated driver who tries to enter and much later, tries to find his car. The foundation staff is extremely helpful and when times are trying, a situation occurs that brings everything back into perspective. For example, "when a person who is showing signs of stress, and is struggling to operate the car park card vending machine or the delight of a young child putting the coins into the machine to receive the card and you discover both persons have just come from chemotherapy treatment." Life, then takes on more meaning!

Nonetheless, The National Heart Foundation of Australia is to be highly commended for the amount of informative information that exists for patients in the way of books, brochures and pamphlets. I know I was facing an information overload but it did not stop me from further researching into the problems of an aortic valve replacement and the necessity for a triple coronary artery bypass graft.

In addition, I need to thank all the drug companies that have provided the research and the drugs that create an all important health zone. However, I still ponder the question, "Are we absorbing too many drugs into our system?"

To my sisters and brother, Patricia, Peter, Juanita and my brother-in-law John who spent two weeks with us in paradise, and fulfilled their dream of seeing a healthy person rather than one of frailty. I thank them for their motherly love, their sense of humour and their caring inspirational support. They took the time to read my manuscript, discussed the chapter of events and offered their suggestions. To my son Darren and Danni, their enthusiasm, support, determination, and their laughter put me on the road to recovery.

On the whole, the foundation of love goes to the gold medalist Nela, my wife, my soul mate, friend and confidant. Her very existence is the springboard that inspires and motivates my life on earth.

Chapter 29
My Medication

The Good! Although my daily dose of medication consists of a potpourri of Allopurinal (zyloprim) that helps prevent gout, Omeprazole that treats and/or prevents ulcers, to Metoprolol that regulates my heartbeat which may decide to do a Latin American salsa dance together with the Atorvastatin tablet and a 100mg aspirin that thins the blood. Occasionally when necessary, I may have to take Colchcine tablets, if under attack by the dreadful gout gremlin.

I cannot stress the importance of taking the tabs on a regular basis and the importance of drinking 6-8 glasses of water to flush out all the toxins that are floating around the system.

Nevertheless, the Atorvastatin tablet that I also partake in the libation for a strong, beating heart has me most intrigued, as it helps to reduce our cholesterol levels. You may remember in Chapter 3 when Dr Challa told me that I needed an aortic valve replacement and a triple by-pass graft. I was amazed by this turn of events and questioned my cholesterol level never thinking that within the very near future I would be lying on an operating table. Why? Because somewhere in my lifetime I may have eaten more saturated fats than I should have! 'Was it my daily intake of cheese that caused this downfall or was it something else, I ponder as I put pen to paper?'

I believe it is necessary to iterate the several types of cholesterol:
- **The Good** (HDL) Cholesterol – HDL (good) cholesterol doesn't get deposited in the arteries but is broken down by the liver. Some experts believe that HDL can actually remove cholesterol from the lining of the arteries.
- **The Bad** (LDL) Cholesterol – LDL (bad) cholesterol causes fatty deposits in the inner ling of arteries, which can increase your risk of heart disease.
- **The Ugly** (Triglyceride) – Triglyceride (TG) pronounced 'try-gliss-a-ride', is another type of blood fat. High triglyceride levels

often mean you're good (HDL) cholesterol levels are low. High triglyceride combined with high bad (LDL) cholesterol can further increase heart risk. (Lipitor atorvastatin –www.pfizer.com.au)

Now that you fully understand the medical jargon; for us mere mortals cholesterol is a type of fat that your body needs to make hormones and essential cell components. So, what makes it? It is made by the liver and is present in some types of food. When too much cholesterol is present in the blood, the excess is deposited in arteries, especially the coronary arteries that supply the heart muscle with oxygen. These deposits make coronary arteries narrower – starving the heart of oxygen. This can cause

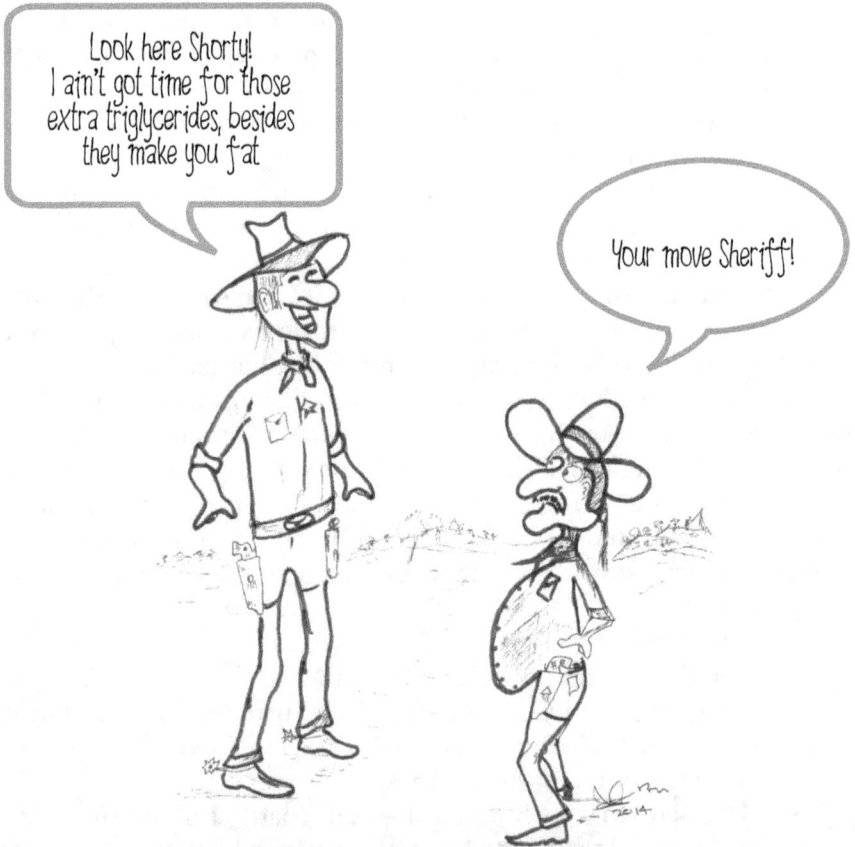

Check your good and bad cholesterol.
Monitor your blood pressure.
See your doctor.

chest pain or angina. Clots form in the artery, block it and causing a heart attack; or they can break off and travel to the brain, causing a stroke.

So, if you have a slight twinge around the heart or if you are feeling unwell don't let it stop you from going to the doctor. Remember I had no symptoms and being physically fit, I went into hospital for a checkup and came out bodily sick!

"The Good, the Bad, the Ugly" - straight out of a spaghetti western. I quickly drew my six-shooter from my well-oiled holster that is tied down to my right thigh. I'm fast, but my reaction is slow when the good HDL calls out, just as the ugly and the bad drew their weapons; I dodge the shots but glancing ricochets off a heavy steel water tank and penetrates my body. Nevertheless, sometime later, a successful operation and I am back on my feet ready to tackle a complete recovery program.

Sometime later, I'm at my kitchen table cleaning and oiling my six-shooter as I think over a range of questions that are like bullets whizzing about in my mind, "What if my cholesterol levels were high? What was the cause? What kind of food was I eating? ' Did I have too much fat in my diet or maybe it was genetically predisposed to having high cholesterol, in other words did it run in my family?'

Likened to a sniper taking aim, having high blood cholesterol is a major risk for heart disease and should not be swept under the carpet and forgotten! Or would you rather a bullet that leads to an unhealthy demise? For me, I'm going to dodge the incoming bullet! "What will you do?"

Yeah! Yeah! What am I going to do? Well for starters I'm going to ensure that the prescribed medicine is taken every day to help reduce my cholesterol. If it is not taken regularly then I'll probably miss out on all the potential benefits that it offers. So what does it actually do? The tablet works by altering the way your body processes fats so that the cholesterol ends up circulating in your bloodstream, and this ultimately protects your heart. However, it is up to you to see your doctor if you are not feeling too well. More-so if, you think the medicine is upsetting your health system.

If you start missing out taking your medications on a regular basis, ask yourself, "Am I protecting my heart as effectively as I should be?' "Do I need to be told later down the track that I now have a heart problem, a problem that could have been easily remedied by having a daily routine in taking the medication?" Remember this is not a chore but a daily ritual that will benefit your health.

After cleaning my pistol, I saddle my horse and ride into town to see the Sheriff, but he is away. I take time to read the Wanted Notices, outside the Sheriff's office. I pull my Stetson down to stop the glare from a burning sun reflecting off the sun baked, dusty road into my eyes. One notice in particular reads, "Most heart disease is preventable. If you already have a heart disease, it's not too late to stop further damage and possibly even reverse it." I know you are going to ask me how? Wouldn't it be nice to think how well you feel and not carrying excess weight around or being frustrated or impatient. The poster explains -

Simply put, you can reduce your heart disease by:
- loving yourself
- eating healthy
- losing weight if you need to
- increasing your activity
- giving up smoking
- being less stressed
- Taking medications every day

If I follow all these healthy habits, what other important benefits may be expected:
- Wouldn't you feel better about yourself?
- Wouldn't you like to reduce the risk of other diseases, such as diabetes, high blood pressure, stroke, other circulation problems and some cancers, such as bowl cancer?

I feel the sun soaking through my clothing but have not finished reading all the Notices. I discover all "fats" are high in energy or kilojoules, and should only be used in small quantities. 'What has fats got to do with my cholesterol,' I thought as I wiped the sweat from my forehead.

"By reducing the saturated fat in your diet you can lower your cholesterol." Why, I thought? Your liver makes most of the cholesterol in your blood from the saturated fat that you eat. So the more saturated fat you eat the more cholesterol your liver produces. Wow! So I need to cut out all those marbled, juicy steaks I eat. Now the penny drops! To reduce my cholesterol levels, all I need to do for it to be effective is to reduce the amount of saturated fat that I eat, but I don't necessarily have to cut out cholesterol-containing foods.

However, it mentions that small quantities of polyunsaturated and monounsaturated fats are good for your health. 'Hmm! Therefore, healthy eating, and reducing the risks to heart disease will see me wearing a gold medal, but will it be me?' I muse as I move to read another piece of information.

A new, healthy lifestyle will give me directions as to the types of food that I will need to say goodbye to or reduce dramatically. Saturated fats are found in animal and vegetable fats like:

fatty meats	sausages	pastries	chips
full-cream dairy foods	crisps	chocolates	biscuits
	cakes	coconut	

Well! Well! Sodium. Looks like I'll have to cut down on my salt intake! How much salt do you use when cooking or having dinner at the table? How much salt do you realize is in cooked or processed food containing high sodium levels? For instance, a moderate level of sodium is less than 400mg/100g yet in some instant noodles or preserved chili paste it is extremely higher. For peace of mind, check the food label but buy products with less than 120mg sodium serving.

If I'm taking in a lot of salt what can I expect health-wise? In a nut-shell there is strong evidence that too much sodium in the diet causes high blood pressure. So what's the choice? Easy, decrease it and be healthy.

Now here's a choice subject! 'How much fibre are you eating? You know that fibre is best known for keeping the bowels working, and a good dose of constipation is not what you really want.' I reflect as drops of sweat trickle down my face. However, some kinds of fibre can also help lower your cholesterol levels. Did you know that increasing the amount of fibre you eat will also help stop you from overeating, as it is very filling? Ok! What type of food should I eat to get more fibre? Try eating a range of fruits, vegetables, cereals, grains, breads, seeds and nuts.

I hear the sound of clip, clop from a horse's hooves, turning around I look up and gaze into the tired eyes of the sheriff. "Howdy, sheriff, been riding long?" I ask, looking at his sweat, soaked shirt. 'Yeah' Lou, been investigating that theft of fresh food that was supposed to be on the wagon last weekend, I followed the tracks to the canyon but lost them among the granite rocks, the robbers left no other signs, except for empty food packages." I found a parcel addressed to the Doc. "It was labeled cholesterol medicine, it's a mystery? I'll ask the Doc about it," he said. "What kind of food did they take?" I asked. The labels indicate that there were dried nuts of different varieties, fruit, grains and apples," the sheriff answered.

I said, "Let's eat and you can wash down some of that dust out of your throat." "Okay! But give me 15 minutes to wash some of this grime off and put on a clean shirt; I sure am thirsty, I'll meet you over at the diner," he replied wearily.

Sitting down at the table, I order soup and crackers but the sheriff decided on a large steak with lots of fat running through it, lots of potatoes covered in a lake of salty gravy. I told him I had read most of the Notices outside his office and that he should do the same because it would provide some answers as to why he is putting on extra weight. He needed to look at the large poster that gave tips for healthy eating.

He said, "I've glanced at them, but I wasn't interested." I looked at him and shook my head, "You really need to read them and to take off that weight otherwise you are going to have a health problem. You don't have to starve yourself, you can make good food choices that have less fat and sugar; gradually your waist will reappear," I said. He answered with a sigh, "I guess you're right, trying to get on my horse or riding is becoming more difficult each day, so I'll go and see the doctor later this afternoon and also find out about that package I found!" I suppose I need to tell myself, lose it or wear it otherwise I'm heading for trouble down the track.

"You know that smoking doesn't help you, it's time to quit but it's your choice. However, if you leave it too late then you only have yourself to blame for your health problems in the future." I said. The sheriff looked at his cigarette and dropped it into the empty bottle of beer he had been drinking. "I guess so, that's it! I'm going to turn over a new leaf! So with your support I'll start a new healthy lifestyle, if you help me with a health program!" he replied. Looking at him, I said, "You are my friend and how can I refuse a friend from choosing a new healthy lifestyle."

After lunch, I said, "We would meet later on in the week and talk about all the other information on the notice-board." I untied my wonderful horse "Star," from the hitching rail, mounted, straightened my Stetson and rode off to my ranch that was built beside a fast running river some 10 kilometers away,.

During the ride home, I thought about the notice on diabetes and the possibility of the sheriff having it, because he was really overweight. I hated to think that he may develop other health problems such as hypertension, stroke, kidney failure and limb amputation. It seems that people with diabetes do not convert blood sugar (glucose) into energy effectively, either because they do not produce enough insulin (type 1 diabetes) or because their insulin no longer works properly (type 2 diabetes).

Well it gets back to whether you want to be sick or healthy. It's your choice, what comes first your health or sickness? I know diabetes cannot be cured but it can be controlled with healthy eating. So what is the secret? To achieve good diabetes control it is important to eat a moderate amount of carbohydrates, cut down on fat, especially saturated fats, eat moderate amounts of protein and in addition I need to choose foods low in salt and to drink plenty of water and to limit my intake of alcohol.

A slight cool breeze is coming off the river and the clip clop of the horses hooves resonate through the air as I near home. I know that I have a lot of changes make to achieve a healthy lifestyle. It is time to put thoughts into action rather than sit around waiting for a miracle to happen!

Oh! I can see smoke coming from the ranch house chimney. The cook has been busy but he doesn't know about my health plan. I don't want to hurt his feelings, but I'll have to be honest with him and explain the program to him. Maybe he will also see the value of good healthy eating and this will show in future menus!

In the meantime, I'll need to spend time organizing the new work schedules, from fixing the fence posts to replacing the fence wire, to the dust mustering of cattle and the branding of the young calves to repairing the windmill amongst many other jobs before I can ride into town to see the sheriff once more.

Chapter 30
Laminated Wallet-size Medication Information

Name: _____

Address: _____

_____

City: _____ State: ____ Post Code: _____

DOB: _____

Doctor: _____

Address: _____

_____

City: _____ State: ____ Post Code _____

Phone: _____

Present Medication:

1.

2.

3.

4.

5.

Cardiac Surgeon: _____

Type of Operation: _____

Date of Operation: _____

Name of Hospital: _____

Blood Type: _____

Making a laminated, wallet-size, medication information data card is invaluable. When the Doctor asks you what type of tablets you take; you don't have to say, 'I think it is a yellow one!' I know I take a brown and a pink one.' You now have all the information at your fingertips.

Remember to update it as your medication changes.

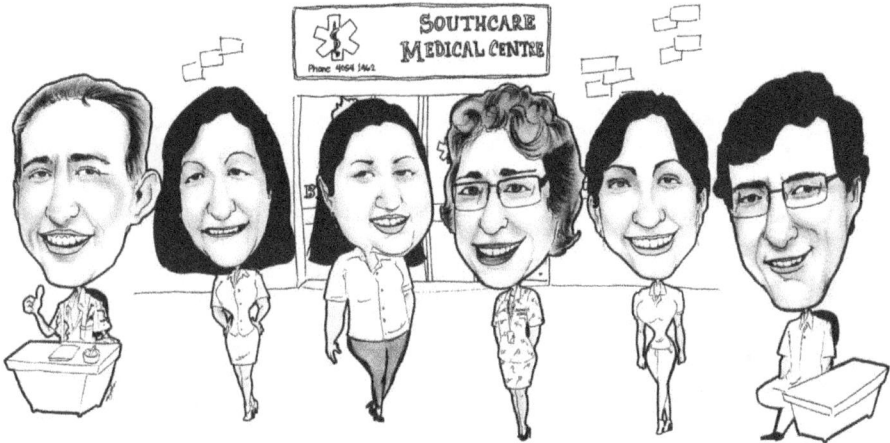

The Go to see people

The Day of
My Aneurysm

Are you a walking time bomb?

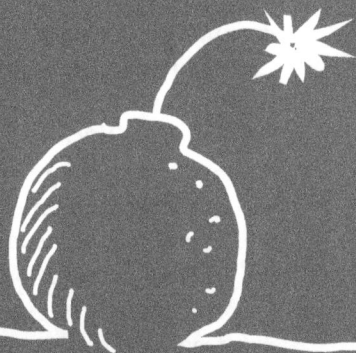

PRELUDE

Many men love machinery - especially cars. They marvel at how they perform quietly and efficiently. The car's systems: hydraulics, battery, cooling, fuel, and air conditioning, all mesh together to create a smooth driving experience. Men who love their cars, diligently care for them, and know that maintenance is the key to longevity and a good trade-in price! They are thorough, and check and re-check to keep the precious car in top condition.

Many men are unaware of another machine in their lives – their body. The human body is a similar mesh of systems, working together to deliver a healthy life. The body has a circulatory system. It has a breathing system. It has a digestive system. It has a cooling system. It has a brain/sensory system. And more...

It is the most advanced, integrated system on the planet.

It is a machine!

But many men ignore this machine or take it for granted. They do not treat it with the same care and respect they shower on their cars. As they grow older, many men just put up with the signals their bodies send, and grumble about slowing down physically.

Unfortunately many men add to their body problems. They smoke, consume too much alcohol, eat unwisely, are inactive, and completely ignore sound advice that filters into all our lives through TV, the press and word-of-mouth. This lack of care can result in dire consequences for this human machine.

While I have taken a focus on men and machinery, it doesn't mean I don't realise that many women also allow a focus on family and work responsibilities to be all-consuming, and for the result to be the same – the importance of caring for the body, being de-prioritised.

Loury's medical journey supports the moral of the analogy we have established for you - "Take care of yourself." Know and respect your body and its systems; know and implement healthy behaviors; and maintain a positive attitude and outlook on life, and be there for others in times of adversity.

We urge you to read Loury's experiences, and take on the message, that prevention is better than cure. If it is your lot to experience similar surgery, Loury's book gives clear and concise details on every step, from admission to recovery. It is in your interest to read it.

Loury's nature, determination and willingness to help others is a mark of the man we know as our friend.

Ron Clarke and Ngaire Tagney
26th February 2014

Chapter 1
A Walking Time Bomb!

What is an aneurysm? The majority of people would say it is a clot that occurs in a blood vessel in the brain. Correct, but did you know that...? Nevertheless, are you a walking time-bomb?

However, let me digress for a moment to the 27th July 2012, when my wife Nela and I flew to Bangkok to attend a double birthday celebration and to visit Thailand's Adenium (desert rose) nurseries. It was not amidst the hectic queues of the thousands passing through Bangkok's passport control, nor was it due to the Dolly Parton look-alike thrusting her breasts into my face at the famous Tiffany Boys Show in Pattaya or living my dream of walking and playing with the tigers at the Tiger Temple at Kanchanaburi. It was at the insistence of our friend, Nisy, to take me to the Bangkok Chao Phya Private Hospital because of the bout of food poisoning that had been bugging (excuse the pun!) me for one week.

In the course of examining my abdomen with her gentle fingers, the doctor of the gastrointestinal unit explained to Nisy that I had to be extra careful of the aneurysm and be wary of knocking or falling over as it could rupture! Aneurysm! What aneurysm? "Is there a blood clot taking a trip to my brain?" I asked hoarsely. "No!" the good Doctor smiled and assured me by taking both my hands and guiding them onto my abdomen where I felt the pulsating of my heart! Heart! Did it drop? "No! No! Your heart hasn't dropped," she laughed. "That is the symptom of an abdominal aortic aneurysm (AAA)," she replied sauntering back to her desk.

Unfortunately, the good Doctor did not mention that lifting heavy things could cause a rupture of the aorta. Here I am lifting heavy bags into taxis, buses and throwing them onto airport scales, but the *piece de resistance* was on our arrival back in Sydney in August. After lifting the bags onto the trolley and pushing it about thirty meters, I noticed one wheel had decided to misbehave and this caused a tremendous amount of exertion on my part. By the time we reached the quarantine inspection table I was absolutely buggered! Fortunately we got the green light to leave and to move to the transit baggage section for our bags to be loaded onto our Cairns flight.

Arriving back in Cairns, I promptly made an appointment to see Dr Derrick Coetzee of South Care Medical Centre, who requested a CT scan at the North Queensland X-ray Services. On 24th August 2012 the result indicated an Abdominal Aortic Aneurysm (AAA) discovered deep within the chasm of my abdomen. A referral letter was sent to the Vascular Unit at the Cairns Base Hospital on Tuesday 28th August and the following day I received a telephone call, to advise me that I had an appointment with the surgeon Dr. Christina Steffen, on 10th September, 2012 to discuss the aneurysm and the possibility of a surgical operation.

Take a hot dog, stand it in a vertical position and completely squash a delightful hamburger and place it behind the red hot dog that forms the aorta with the hamburger being your aneurysm. A simple technical explanation of my aneurysm that it is 8.2 cms in transverse diameter, the maximum is 5.5cms. Now that is clear as mud! A conference with the doctor, the registrar and others eyeballing my x-ray of the now famous aneurysm proved to be positive. With those long awaited words Dr. Steffen said, "I'm free! I'm free! We'll pencil in the date for his operation for Wednesday 24th October, 2012."

Research indicates that the aorta is the largest artery in the body. The part of the aorta that carries blood from your heart through to your abdomen then splits itself into the iliac arteries that supply your legs is called the abdominal aorta. Various smaller arteries also branch off the aorta at several points to carry blood to various organs and to other parts of the body. An aneurysm occurs when a weakened part of a blood vessel expands like a balloon. During the expansion the vessel becomes thinner and weakens, and there is a risk it will open or rupture creating a life-threatening condition. Ironically, the AAA is often found when tests are done for an unrelated problem. If the aneurysm is large enough it can be felt by the doctor when you are lying down, as was the case when mine was discovered in Thailand.

I was reasonably physically fit and did not know that anything was wrong! However, it was after the diagnosis in Cairns that I discovered that some previous experiences pointed to my abdominal aortic aneurysm. The major one was the pulsating feeling in my abdomen and unexplained backaches, the latter, I put down to building and working in the garden. This problem often appears especially in men, who are over 60 years old. So if you detect a pulsating feeling in your abdomen, check with your doctor.

It's Thursday 18th October, and I have just completed my morning stint with the Cairns Cardiac Rehabilitation Unit (CRU) that has relocated to the Cairns North Community Health Centre.

The staff and volunteers, of which I am one, help new and old patients come alive during their rehab individual exercise and education program. The volunteers are a zany bunch of former heart patients who can provide helpful information; we sing and go through our soft shoe shuffle routine. We make it a happy event! However, after my last patient has completed his exercise program, I move swiftly to my hot and trusty steed that is waiting outside in the car park. I motor to the Cairns Base Hospital (CBH) to attend my pre-admission assessment and the information overload for my forthcoming trip to the bright lights of the operating theatre.

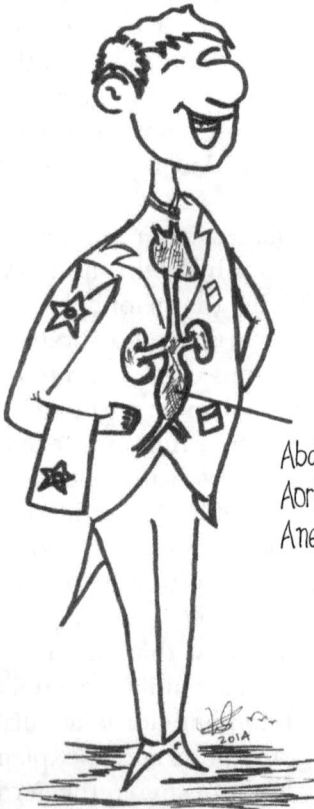

Abdominal
Aortic
Aneurysm

But, I had no ideal I had no symptoms and yet...!

Instead of going down the main drag and facing the numerous traffic lights I take the many side streets and the several round-about's that confuse locals and tourists alike. But it is the magnificent drive along the Esplanade and the view out to sea that has a calming effect upon one's senses. Ten minutes later I arrive at the hospital car park only to find it full. So for the next 15 minutes I roam around until once more I arrive at the car park and find a vacant spot. I expect to be at the hospital for four hours and after hunting around inside my trouser pocket I finally find the elusive two dollars and sixty cents that will give me the time required. Walking across the road to the hospital entrance I gasp as my senses are smothered in cigarette smoke from patients who are unable to realize the health risks that they will endure. The exhaled passive smoke that engulfs the non-smokers is equally dangerous. I wonder why *smokers insist on making the manufacturers rich to the extent of making themselves sick.*

My first stop is the vampires den. I carefully placed my 'request for blood form' into the yawning cave opening of the door and waited for my name to be called. I'm third down the track and I think of the young baby ahead of me, but then it is my turn. A tightening of the strap around my huge bicep ensures that a decent vein is found and the inevitable thrust of the needle sees a river of blood pour forth into the catchment of the vampire's flask. She grins and allows me to leave after placing a swab over the minute pin pri... Oops! Puncture!

I walk to the elevator and ascend to the first floor and make my presence felt by taking a number from a machine that is hidden behind the back of the hospital foundation volunteer. Several minutes lapse and like a lotto winner I proceed to window one, where I am told to sit within the waiting zone of the vascular unit. Shortly, my name is called and a nurse arrives with a questionnaire form that has to be completed for the Registrars to review. Duly completed and the Forms handed over, I sit amongst the small waiting crowd until once more, I am called and beckoned into a small office to converse with Anne, the Unit Nurse. Her cheerfulness puts me at ease, although I am relaxed as I have continually practiced my deep breathing exercise of getting my 'one point,' and extending my Ki. Anne takes me through the general information booklet for patients undergoing vascular surgery at the Cairns Base Hospital

Twenty minutes later, and once more in the waiting room, I am again called and I go for an ECG. Gazing around, 'I've been here before and you took my ECG in 2009, I uttered to the nurse, and if I am not mistaken you come from Indonesia!' I said. In reply, she said, "Wow! You have a great memory!" I have, but the years have diminished this skill and I often ask myself, 'What did I come in here for? I think for a minute or two and the answer hits my brainwaves and I locate the item of discovery!' But then, it is back to the waiting room.

Taking pen to newspaper, i.e. the crossword, I settle down to wait for my next meeting, 10 minutes later I face a memory blank but the dulcet tones from a mysterious voice calls my name. Standing, the voice introduces himself as Skip Townsend; "I'm going to be your anesthetist," he said.

Settling down with ease, Skip goes through the procedures for my operation. You will have two IV lines, one arterial line, a general anesthetic, a central venous line and an epidural injection into the back that will help against the pain factor. This will enable you to sleep comfortably. You will be in the Intensive Care Unit (ICU) overnight but we may extend the time, if you become a 'bleeder' and require more blood throughout the operation. More information, more questions, alleviates the mind!

Skip needs to ensure that my previous blood request will also provide for cross-matching other types for the operation, hence a second trip to see the delightful vampires. Telephone conversations allay any problems with the request and I head back to the vascular unit. My next meet is with the registrar who assists the surgeon.

The recording starts again and I am ushered into the interviewing room with the young, refreshing Dr Zoe, who provides additional information about my operation to be held on Wednesday, 24th October! She advises that I will need to call the Day Surgery Unit the day before, to ascertain whether it will be a morning or afternoon surgical operation. Back to the waiting room!

Dr Townsend completes a request form for an echocardiogram (ECG) to be administered before my operation takes place. The following Monday morning, I am told that my appointment is for an ECG at 3:00pm that afternoon. I arrive at 2:30pm, ascend to the 3rd floor and go to the Echo reporting office. Alas! No one is in the office! I sit down and read, but the antics of a young, three year old girl holds my attention as she practices her rap dancing, and plays imagination basketball and cricket with her mother. How refreshing!

Time is flying and the sonographer asks me if I am to have an echo and did I go to the front counter? Sheepishly, I said, "What an idiot, I am! I went to the wrong office." Fortunately, the receptionist was still in the main office and I was able to complete the necessary information.

The young, attractive, blonde Azra who hails from Bosnia discovered that my heart was alive as it swished its way through the instrumentation of technology. We had a delightful conversation throughout the monitoring of the echocardiogram machine. All too soon it ended and I was taking the elevator back to the ground floor and walking out into the bright sunshine to the car park. Putting all the windows down in the furnace of my car I relished the sea breeze that brought the temperature down and allowed me to drive home in comfort.

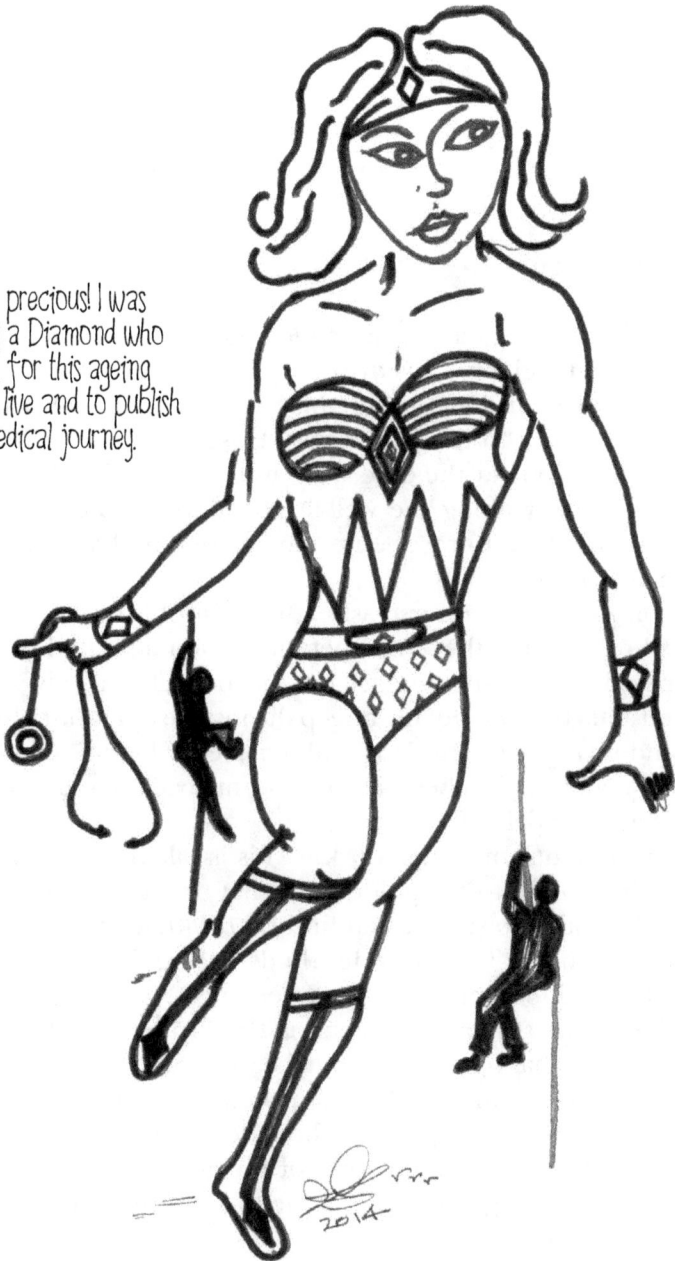

Life is precious! I was saved by a Diamond who fought for this ageing person to live and to publish his medical journey.

Chapter 2
A Glimmer of Light

The Operation

This is the big day, the 24th October 2012. Gary Schofield our good friend and neighbour has driven up behind my white Pajero 4x4 in his blue, Suburu Forester, blowing his horn. He waited in readiness, to take both Nela and I to the Cairns Base Hospital. Arriving at the entrance I take a good look at the blue skies and the serenity of the ocean before I make my way along the well-lit corridors. I enter the realms of the Admission Office to receive my paper work, and then take the elevator to the day surgical unit.

On Admission a nurse asks a final list of questions to ensure that I am who I am, for the AAA operation. I am admitted to the Ward and prepared by the aneasthetist for theatre. That involves giving me an anaesthetic that will put me asleep during the operation. Imagine waking up and saying, 'Yo! Ho! Ho! And a barrel of blood!' Oh, God the pain! But a small tube has been inserted in my back that carries the epidural that waves off pain after surgery.

What about my water works? This is taken care of with a catheter, being inserted into the golden orb that drains the royal fluid from my body. Hurrah! No stone is left unturned with a drip being placed into a vein in my neck. That provides fluids during the operation and also to monitor my blood pressure measurements.

Well! The suspense deepens as Dr Christine Steffen and her trusty surgical team has opened up a much larger crevasse below the breastbone from the edge of the old 2009 archaeological site. Her ever steady hand guides the scalpel, deep within the widening crevasse, allowing the team to abseil into the deeper depths of the abdomen in their quest to find the golden hotdog and the squashed hamburger that defines the aorta and the aneurysm.

Reaching the outskirts of the granite navel and not wishing to dull the cutting edge of the scalpel the team decided to make a small detour around the navel and back to the central median line then to the level of the hipline. Entering into the coils of intestines, they finally arrive at the sleeping serpentine of the bowel ducting. Carefully, they move this serpentine out of its habitat and onto the outer side of my stomach, and from an unobstructed view they look into a well of claret.

Their prize is hidden, but as they search, the pool of claret decreases and they see a glimmer of light that produces a golden halo around the hotdog and the hamburger. There is no time to give each other their 'high five' as a cause for celebration, because it is now vital to clamp both ends of the aorta before they can proceed to the next step.

From all accounts the hotdog is now sliced open and through the amazing science of creativity an artificial blood vessel made of Dacron replaces the hamburger aneurysm. The flaps encase this man-made miracle like a cocoon, and sewn with the finest of stitching, delicate fingers ensure that all is stable. The reality of the situation cannot escape me as this is done within a pool of blood. Alas! The release of the clamps, the blood flows, but disaster strikes as a pinprick appears and I have become a bleeder. I was told this may occur during my pre-admission assessment, but who could predict this unforeseen situation. This is life threatening! Take an inner tube, and look for a puncture hole by immersing it in water. Bubbles appear and you have discovered it. Now throw in some red dye and try to repair it under water!

The blood consists of liquid and three kinds of solid particles called formed elements. These are liquid plasma, red blood cells, white blood cells and platelets. Platelets are disc-like structures that help prevent bleeding from damaged blood cells, in other words the platelets seal broken vessels by forming a clot. In this instance, the clot did not occur! (World Book Encyclopedia, 1989, USA)

The team must find the cause of the bleeding. However, this is not the time for panic nor is there a need for haste. There is a need to put together the years of experience of the team and a leader who can make decisions, be cool under extreme circumstances, and be in the zone that she can feel every nuance of the blood vessels beneath her fingers. This delicate operation will lead to a successful outcome. More-so as the pin hole was very close to the kidneys and this increased the gravity of the situation, under trying conditions.

What was expected to take between two to three hours has taken six hours. The extra hours have completely drained the team of energy. They are tired. Nevertheless they have sutured and stemmed the flow of blood that has taken some 22 bags of donor cross-matched blood to ensure that I am alive to write the final chapter to Santa's Cardio Rehab Boot Camp and The Day of My Aneurysm. The wounds are closed and like several sheets of paper, not one but 42 staple clips adorn my 75 year old six-pack physique that has now wrinkled. Those once admired AB's resemble my mother's old washboard of yesteryear!

Intensive Care Unit

I am now in the Intensive Care Unit (ICU). My wife Nela and my son Darren have arrived and are taken aback at my appearance. Both are teary. My whole body is swollen I have grown out of proportion. Darren in a hoarse voice asks, 'what has happened to Dad?' Whispering, Nela replies, "It must be due to all the blood loss!" My eyes have glazed over and I am unable to speak as I still have a metallic object in my throat and I am still hooked up to the various life lines.

I have no pain. The epidural has done wonders, but the drugs have me in a world of hallucination. I can see reruns of TV programs and watch basketball films from the late 40's. I hear distinct voices of friends I know. I clearly hear my good friend Bill Lee Long, speaking to a female nurse and of two Chinese boys playing on hand drums! However, as I vainly try opening my eyes I find I am again hallucinating!

This is my second day, and I am still hooked up on the breathing machine. I still cannot talk, yet my eyes can now focus on faces and their movement around me. I will continue being drip fed until such time as the serpentine within the body copes with fluids taken in through the mouth as the unpleasantness of bodily activity has stopped for the interim.

Day three, and the physiotherapist arrived to help me back on my feet, but it is fruitless. I am unable to stand, let alone walk. I need to shower and the only way now, is to be placed in a hoist like a sack of rice in a saddle bag and wheeled from ICU 13 along the corridors to the bathroom. After completing my ablutions, a wheelchair comes to my aid and I am able to return to my bedside. Another day and I finally leave the ICU, and moved to the day surgery ward.

Day Surgery Ward

I have a room and a toilet and a shower. The toilet is so close but as I am unable to walk, let alone get out of bed I unfortunately suffer six mishaps. That was a source of embarrassment to my ego. However, these delicate moments are outweighed by the dedication of the group of fine, young nurses who are following their pathway of dreams in helping and caring for those in need. To Madeline, Christine, Jessica, Alana, Meagan and to the rest of the support group I salute and thank you.

A day later and a young physiotherapist arrived with his assistant to put me through some exercises, eventually with some effort I was able get out of bed and walk with the aid of a metal frame walker. Later, he was checking out my legs on the bed and wondered how I had an unusual scar on my inner, left leg. I replied, "It was my battle scar, when I was a freelance journalist in Afghanistan." Unfortunately, I could not keep a straight face and laughed. The scar was from my 2009 operation.

Doctor Steffen and her entourage arrived and were quite happy with the healing of my wound that had some 42 staples holding the folded skin together. She said, "We are going to remove the catheter to see if you can pee within a six hour period!" What can I say except say; *your wish is my command.*

The catheter was duly removed, and I waited, and I waited for the expected feeling of, 'it's time to pee!' Unfortunately, this did not occur and after seven hours. I spoke to the nurse, who in turn contacted a doctor who came to investigate the problem and to see if I needed the catheter returned to release the dam that was building within me.

"Nurse, have a look at the pipe line, it's retracted inwards. I think he's circumcised!" "Hey, mate are you circumcised?" he asked. In a befuddled state of mind, I said, "Yes." "ARE you sure you are circumcised?" he again asked. "Yes! Yes!" I replied. But once more he asked the same question and tiredly I replied, "Yes!" Having been assured that I was really circumcised, the doctor rejoined the catheter to the be-jeweled golden orb and within seconds, the royal fluid from the pierced dam, gushes into the holding tank. Ahh! What relief! A couple of days later the catheter is removed, once more with great success, as the function of peeing becomes a routine of relief.

My energy level is low and my appetite cannot take in the smell of the hospital gourmet food.

My golden jewels have swollen to the size of emu eggs but the royal golden orb has once again receded into obscurity. I call upon Dr Harris, a member of the surgical team who visits me each day. I tell him of my problem! Putting on a pair of royal blue (the Queens Diamond Jubilee), anti-bacterial gloves, he examines by prodding, pulling and stretching until the pipeline appears. He advises, "If it disappears again, then you have to prod, pull and stretch for it to reappear." 'But how many times will I need to prod, pull and stretch before I go blind?' I wonder!

The ward team leader must have been beside herself, when an entourage lead by Mandi, Anita, Jacquie, Bill, Anne and Nick from the Cardiac Rehabilitation Unit infiltrated my room. It was noisy with laughter and I am grateful for their presence and friendship. Likewise, I am also grateful to Anne Chirio, Volunteer Coordinator for the Hospital Foundation and my other numerous friends who motivated me by cheering me and raising my spirits high for a speedy recover.

It's Saturday, 3rd November 2012. Dr's Steffen and Thram are doing their hospital rounds. They have checked my wound and are satisfied that it is healing thoroughly. Both agree that I could go home that morning. Taken aback for a few minutes, I finally agree that my home environment would do wonders for my recovery. Dr Thram advises that I should not be doing any golf swings, but I can do bicep curls and shoulder stretches and can carry the combined weight of two telephone directories.

The nurse tried to contact my wife, Nela, but she and our dear friend Gary Schofield were already on their way to the hospital.

I've shaved, showered, and the nurse has applied the final dressings to my battle scar wound. I have dressed, and opened my Lee Child, the author of the popular Jack Reacher thriller novel series, called "The Hard Way", I became engrossed as I waited for Nela to arrive. Upon her arrival, I surprised her by saying, "The nurse has been trying to contact you because I'm being discharged once the paperwork has been completed." She was taken aback as she was not prepared for this sudden decision for my discharge. The nurse gave us a two separate telephone numbers to call for home assistance, as she was unable to contact the Social Worker.

Gary has dropped Nela off at the hospital and was not due back until later in the afternoon. We were lucky to contact our friend, Mayet, who came and picked us up at 12:30pm. After a brief stopover at the Raintree's supermarket to buy fresh bread rolls and salad for lunch, she then drove us home.

Chapter 3
Recovery Blues

Clear, Blue skies above and we arrived at our castle that nestles at the foothills of a green, tree covered, mountain range that is dotted with outcrops of granite rock, formed millions of years ago during the mountain's uplift,

Alighting from Mayet's dark blue, Ford Escape, I shuffle through the front gate and we are met by a happy tongue licking, black Rottweiler-Doberman cross, named Bella. In those moments of joy I contemplate my rash decision of being discharged from the Cairns Base Hospital today, especially after spending ten days there from a near death experience.

"Was it a rash decision," I asked myself. More-so, as I was still weak. The lack of appetite had depleted my energy levels. I was still suffering from minor bouts of diarrhea and to make matters worse my family jewels were still largely swollen!

Had I thought about the pressure I was going to put on my wife, Nela, in caring for me, especially since she had her own health issues to worry about? Did I really think about other problems that may arise, like going to the Doctors? Who was going to drive me there? How were we going to get our groceries etc.?

My reasoning behind the decision was that my recovery would be much faster within my familiar, home surroundings. However, the question that begs answering is, "How long will it take me to get back to normal?"

This answer lies in my attitude. "If I'm not in control of things, don't stress out." This is my mantra. Nevertheless, I am in control of my recovery! Now is not the time to think, "what if...!" Nor is it the time to dwell amongst the seeds of self-pity of, "why me? What have I done to deserve this problem?" No! This is the time for action, to map out my rehabilitation program. Unfortunately, I did not receive anything upon my discharge concerning this aspect of my hospitalization treatment. I must rely on the experience from my 2009 heart operation and what I have gleaned in my work as a volunteer with the Cardiac Rehabilitation Unit for my recovery to be successful!

I begin the next three weeks with a ten day course of amoxicillin tablets that will ward off possible infections within my body. Unfortunately, they strongly react with my bodily movements in the form of the dreaded diarrhea that further depletes my energy level. Added to this mix is a bout of reflux that has decided to join the forces of evil!

An appointment with Dr Coetzee sees the removal of the last of the 42 staples that has held the crevasse together. There is no seepage of blood and the wound is healing quite well! He has recommended that I take gastrolyte that will help me replace the electrolytes lost due to my bouts of diarrhea and other dehydrating conditions; also I need to take Inner Health Plus and Zinc supplement tablets that will support the immune system, gives anti-oxidant protection and provides for healthy skin support. They worked wonders! (N.B. Check with your own Doctor before use!)

My throat was still sore from the operation and chewing food was rather difficult. Hence, in those three weeks all I wanted to eat was soup with noodles, mince with rice and soft, stir fried vegetables, etc.

Like a pregnant woman I had sudden food urges! A point in time was my desire to have Campbell's chicken noodle soup. I asked Nela if we had any in the pantry. In reply, she said, "No," but we had other brands and also we have frozen potato and leek soup or pumpkin soup in the freezer. We often make large batches of soup and freeze them in the large, plastic Yoplait yogurt containers. But for this 75 year old, my heart's desire was not on the menu! Nela decided to walk over to Sue and Gary's house to see if they had any in stock in their huge pantry. But again the cupboard was bare.

Kind-hearted Gary said, "Look the Stockland supermarkets are still open. So I'll drive down and buy this miracle soup for Loury." Nela in reply said, "Don't bother. I'll just defrost some pumpkin soup for him." Gary was adamant, and said, "It's no bother and I'll be back in a flash!"

Time elapsed and Sue said, "I wonder where Gary is, he said he would be back in a flash?" It's taking him a long time. Ten minutes later, he drives into his garage. The car door is gently closed and he walks into the family room.

"What took you so long?" asked Sue. "Well, I went around to each of the supermarkets and could not find this miracle brand soup that will fulfill Loury's heart's desire! So I went to the local convenient store, but de nada! Then I decided to go to our local Chinese Takeaway and

Restaurant and ordered the chicken noodle soup. So here it is! Piping Hot! I'm sure Loury will enjoy it!"

Enjoy it, I did! The noodles slipped down my raspy, sore throat and I made sure that I kept some for the next day's lunch.

It is Saturday 17th November, and our good friends Gloria, Liza and Nellie have cooked up several dishes of Filipino cuisine and have invited themselves over for lunch, and to see how I was progressing. Two, large servings indicated how much I enjoyed the lunch and the sweet, caramel pudding called leche plan. I knew I was on the way to a healthy recovery, but this thought came too soon!

The next morning I was up at 6:30 and went through my usual routine of starting the day fresh. I had taken my daily consumption of prescribed medicine tablets, switched on the TV and sat down to watch the 7:00 o'clock 'Sunrise' news. Suddenly, I felt unwell, became very clammy and I was uncomfortable around the chest region.

In a hoarse voice, I called Nela who was tendering her exotic desert rose babies. I think she was rather annoyed about coming in, until I told her to ring triple 0. Her face rapidly changed to show concern! I said, "I'm really clammy and it feels like two screws are tightening around my chest!" Contacting 000 she asks for an ambulance and answers all the questions being asked by the operator, who assured her that a Paramedic would be there in 10 minutes and to make sure that he had access through the front door upon his arrival.

By the time Paramedic Gavin had arrived the pain had increased and I was sweating profusely, saturating my tee shirt with perspiration. In the meantime, while I was answering Gavin's questions, he was reassuring me that my heart was OK and that I was probably having post operation pain. He had me wired up to the ECG machine and had taken my blood pressure. Positive results were printed on his high tech machine.

"Hello! Hello!" Echoed back to the family room! "Come in!" Nela and Gavin yelled. Kevin and Nadine of the Smithfield Ambulance Service entered my view of sight. Gavin explains what has happened to date. Kevin asks if the pain still exists and to give it a rating from 0 to 10. I told them it was an eight with the pain getting worse. The three of them conferred and they decided to give me a small amount of morphine to alleviate the pain. After a minute or two it began to subside.

The three of them decided that I should be taken to the Cairns Base Hospital for further observation. Entering the ambulance I am given another small dosage that lowers the pain level somewhat slightly, but it is still there by the time we reach the hospital and I am readmitted.

I cannot speak highly enough of the paramedics and their modern chariots of life. They work long hours and often forgo their meals whilst attending to their patients. Their actions should be an inspiration to all who come in contact with them.

My day long stay in the triage was an eye-opener. Doctors and nurses were like butterflies as they flit from one patient to another without haste, to watch-over, question, take blood samples, and send them for x-rays, to observe and to collate their findings so that the next shift of personnel knew exactly what was wrong with each patient.

Their efforts are beyond reproach and to those patients who complain about the service, the lack of a bed and the 3x3 metre bed space need to reflect on the work of the triage doctors, nurses and support staff do during their rostered hours of work. Bed and bed spacing are at a premium. This will never change as populations grow. Patients cannot be churned out on conveyor belts, although at times it may have had this effect when one patient was discharged and in a matter of minutes the space was filled as a new patient was wheeled into the triage.

I await the results of my 2nd blood test and should it be negative in all aspects I will be discharged by 4:30 p.m. Dr Harris who was a member of the surgical team during my operation is wearing another hat as the medical officer in the triage. He has told me that he will schedule me for a stress test in two weeks time to ensure nothing unforeseen is playing up with my heart.

Having the green light, I am given my discharge and was asked to leave the confines of the triage. I padded bare-footed, out to the emergency waiting room, to await Nela's arrival with my shoes and a tee shirt that would replace the extra-large, blue pyjama top that was given to me on arrival. Our sudden departure from the house caught us unprepared for the return to the hospital.

It was well past five o'clock when both Darren and Nela arrived to take me home.

Although I spent nearly eight hours in the triage and taking up valuable bed space, I was gratified by the care taken by the triage team continually reassuring me that I was okay during those hours of recovery.

Chapter 4
Explosive Devices

The past three weeks had its ups and downs, and looking back, if it wasn't for the discomfort of the situation it would have been hilarious.

For instance, when we sat down to eat our meals at the dining room table; invariably I had only taken a small morsel of food when there was a sudden urge to visit the throne room. Standing, and with Nela showing concern I rushed along the passage way propelled by the rat-a-rat-tat of a bodily machine gun function. These frequent occurrences, caused Nela to cheekily smile and think, "Here he goes again!"

In most cases, a false alarm was flagged. However, on other occasions, from the very depths of an undiscovered Crater Lake volcano, an explosion erupts hurling, in an ever- upward spiral, a burst of methane gas escapes into the enclosed atmosphere of the throne room, enveloping the senses with its poisonous gases. There is no place to run! No place to hide! There is no time to take in a refreshing, deep breath! You gasp and wish you were on some tropical island, soaking in the sunshine other than in the throne room

During my recent visit to the triage, Dr Harris gave me the green light to drive. I decided to make my first foray into the caverns of our Stockland Shopping Centre and drive Nela there to do some shopping. I felt I had recovered from the bad spells of my unfortunate bodily functions.

Driving into the undercover car park gave me that sense of independence and confidence that I needed to undertake some lengthy walking in the Centre. Taking the escalator to the 1st floor I discover an empty trolley that I could use to maintain my balance if and when I needed it.

Slow walking was the order of the morning as I followed the trail left by Nela's wake as she moved from one supermarket to another! On several occasions I was able to sit, relax and watch the multitude walking slowly or in haste; some pulling crying children while others pushing sleeping tots in their pushers, who were oblivious to the sounds around them.

The clock was fast racing towards noon and I was starting to feel peckish! I had asked Nela to go into the supermarket again because I needed to buy some new razors and while I was standing around waiting for her, disaster struck! I had a slight bodily malfunction! I was willing her to hurry up! When she arrived, she saw in my face that something was wrong! Full of embarrassment I told her the problem.

Pushing a trolley load of food, we slowly, ever so slowly, walked back to the escalator, down to the car, unloaded the trolley and drove home. It was an awkward situation and one that I hope will not be repeated.

But then, events shape the world, and my world was soon to be rudely shaken!

All the explosions and the eruptions over the past few weeks may be similar to the joy and laughter of the multitude as they witnessed the noisy fireworks display of the 2013 New Year's Eve festivities on Sydney's famous Harbour Bridge.

Musing over words of yesteryear, I pick up my pen and write, 'Roses are red, and Violets are blue if the constipation doesn't get you. The other will.' But, 'you've got mail,' brings a smile to my face, but, my imaginative mind seeks more, 'this is sent by express mail, unregistered.' This is more than the Big Bang Theory! Little did I know that these thoughts would come back to haunt me in a very short time!

It is Friday, 23rd November 2012. Just one week out from my recent visit to the Triage at the Cairns Base Hospital and for the last three days I have been hit by the all mother of all constipations. Prune juice, Nature's Own, coloxyl with senna tablets have had little effect. Only the day by day explosions eased the pain,

I had decided to hold out for one more day and to see if relief was just around the corner. It's night and I've had a restless sleep. Alas, at 12.30am in the early hours of the morn the pain becomes unbearable when sitting on the throne. But to make matters worse I suddenly found that my golden orb could not pass water and my thoughts returned to the catheter episode whilst I was in hospital!

Gingerly, I waddled from the throne room and aroused Nela from her sleep. She awakes with a fright and asks, "What's wrong?" I tell her my problem and it is time to call triple 000 for their assistance once again. Explaining the situation to the operator and answering the usual, but helpful questions, Nela is told that the paramedics were on their way.

During the wait, we gather our emergency bag of clothing and shoes to take with us, as we did not want to be caught out like we were last time. Some 10 minutes later paramedics Steve and Mick arrive on our doorstep. Having explained the problem to them, they decided that the hospital would best to treat my ailment. However, both said, "Just don't explode in the ambulance!" I assured them that I would try to hold on and, "make sure you don't hit any rough bumps." I replied.

Arriving in familiar surroundings at 1:40am I am wheeled into the pre-admission section. A few minutes later, Steve says, "I just mentioned your triple AAA operation and suddenly you have a bed!" "It's not what you know, it's who you know!" I replied, grimacing with agonizing pain deep within the lower extremities of my rear end!

I transfer myself slowly from the ambulance gurney to the softness of the triage bed. I thank Steve and Mick and both were happy that they did not go over any bumps. Gazing at the bright lights overhead, I did not have to wait long before a young nurse arrives to take my blood pressure. She is soon followed by the rostered medical officer who quizzes me about the constipation situation.

What is about to occur over the next seven hours is a torture that I would not wish upon anybody, let alone my best friends. Ugh!

Not long after the visit from the Registrar, I am confronted by a male nurse who says "This will not hurt you. It is only warm water." Yet in his hand is a plastic bottle, with a 10cm long nozzle! He continues his message of love, by saying "You will need to turn on your side." I can no longer see his face, but I can imagine his torturous smile as he inserts the nozzle all the way into my blocked canal and squeezes with relish the contents of the warm water into the innards of my body. I have just been introduced to the enema treatment!

"How long will I endure this discomfit?" I asked myself. Seconds, then minutes and after one and a half hours, the tormenting pain continues. The progress for stage one of the enema treatment is zero.

The nurse has observed me during the period and she has now decided that torture treatment two must be introduced to conquer the elusive hidden enemy. Like an illusionist, she steps towards me with a grin, it's time for you to imbibe and to send libations to the gods for their understanding and to free you from this not-so delicate malady. So bottoms (excuse the pun) up and indulge in this delightful potion of foul-tasting fluid that we have brewed for you.

I while away the time and contemplate the movements of the doctors, nurses who are observing and talking to patients who require reassurance, medication and the taking of blood samples continuously. The support staff that wheel patients to the X-Ray unit, or moving new patients into bed spaces that have just been vacated. Before long it is approximately 4:00am and my bodily function again registers zero movement!

How agonizing can you get? The Registrar decides that extreme measures are now required and once again I am confronted by the nurse who has arrived with a one litre, blue plastic jug, filled with another brand of foul-tasting fluid! I eye this evil jug and say "You must be joking!" Grinning she replies, "This delightful drop will move mountains and yours is merely a pimple! You need to drink the entire contents of this delightful concoction that I have prepared for you, but finish it in your own time."

I take my first mouthful and lament over the taste of this delightful nectar that is unfit for raising libations to the gods. However, I follow the instructions and pray that this will be my salvation! It is about 6:00am and the Registrar has informed me that I will be moved to another section to be closer to the toilets. Ironically, my present bed is beside the bathroom. I suppose they need the space for the newest of patients?

I am wheeled to this new location. Nela went over to speak to the male nurse who immediately shushes her." Keep your voice down, people are still sleeping!" All she wanted to ask was the location of the throne room. This was duly pointed out to her.

My stomach begins to gurgle and like a pregnant mum, I said, "I think it's time. I need to go right now!" I shuffle with haste, open the door and head for the throne, barely making it; I shudder from the explosion from the weapon of mass destruction. It was the mother of all blasts! Forget about 'you've got mail. It was a 1200 km missile that delivered an express meaning, "your troubles are over!" I had been hanging onto a precipice by my fingers, they slipped and I hurtled to the ground with a gigantic thud. I was overwhelmed by the tremendous feeling I had when suddenly the weight disappeared from my chest region amidst the essence that pervaded my surroundings.

I gathered my thoughts, as I showered, dressed, combed my damp hair and returned to my bed. The ordeal was not over! Suddenly I was suffering the chest pain that I experienced the week before. Nela went and advised the male nurse and explained the situation. He was a little peeved as he was just about to finish his shift and now he had to find the Registrar.

When the Registrar arrived, she assessed the problem and decided to inject a small amount of morphine to ease the pain. She was happy to discharge me but she had to write a discharge letter for my Doctor before we could leave the hospital. By that time the pain had disappeared.

One pleasing note that I can offer to all, is that, as an amateur nuclear scientist I have proven without doubt that the big bang theory did exist, still exists, and will continue to exist throughout the life of mankind!

We eventually caught a taxi home, and after a sleepless night in the triage I decided that I need to have a short nap. Nevertheless, what would we mere mortals do without the dedication, caring and the integrity of a group of fine doctors, nurses, paramedics and their support staff? Once again I salute and thank you.

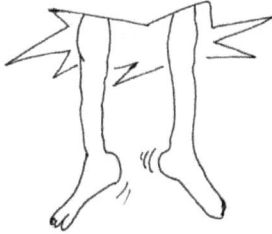

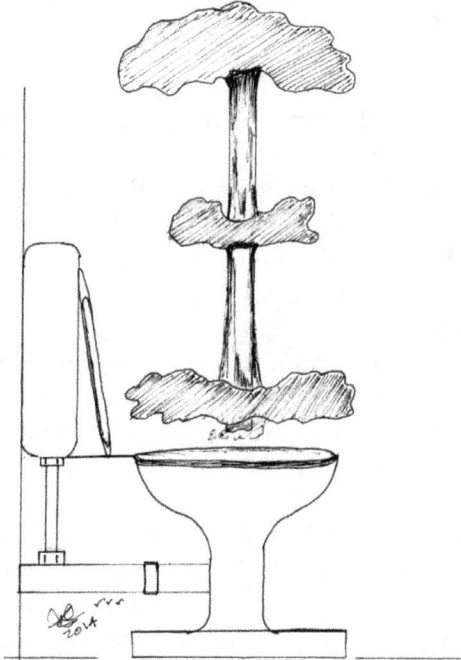

I've just proven that the big bang theory does exist!

Chapter 5
Rehabilitation

From the shuffling along the hospital corridors, to the unsteadiness of starting a 20 minute walk on our 20 metre driveway, then the paced out 220 metre circuit down our close, then pushing myself and stepping out against the clock through power-walking would be the major motivation and the reason towards my recovery

Initially, when I arrived home I pussy-footed along our passageway, but after several days and at the urging of Nela, I ventured outside! I was still lacking energy and breathless during a minor activity. However, her steadying hands provided the balance, as I shuffled to make three circuits of the driveway. By week two, I was slowly walking three circuits each morning and afternoon. Finally I reached my goal of 40 circuits within a time period of 20 minutes. It was time to graduate!

My next step was to pace out a 110metre walk from our driveway to the end of the Close. This gave me a round circuit of 220metres. Taking my time, I cautiously began my walks, especially being mindful of the road camber, small stones and the fallen seed pods from the tree branches overhead; eventually achieving my goal of 10 circuits, and again within a 20 minute time limit.

Over the Christmas period, several of the neighbourhood children asked, "Why are you walking in circles?" I suspect the parents were asking themselves the same question! I stopped and explained that I was recovering from a major surgical operation and that I need to walk to get fit.

Amazingly, after a week I began to walk quite briskly and by the end of the big 10, I was power-walking and perspiring profusely. Wow! I was feeling great! However, it was important for me to do 10 slow circuits of the driveway for my cool down recovery exercise followed up with the usual calf and hamstring stretches, and to prevent dehydration quench my thirst with a bottle of water.

Nela asked, "Why are you carrying that 60 centimetre cane?" In reply,

I said, "Firstly it allows me to practice some of my 'Arnis' stick-fighting skills. I am reminded of my first day, at the Puckupunyal Army Base, along with my best mate, Paul Edwards, and together with many others who had been called up for National Service on 1st January, 1958."

There were several small tables manned by soldiers on the other side of the field. I heard my name called and picking up my bag, I ambled across the field. Suddenly a voice roared out, "You there! This is my parade ground. Don't bloody well amble! March! Left, Right! Left, Right!" So when I find myself slowing down I just remember that tall, ginger-headed Warrant Officer dressed in khaki, long brown socks, dusty brown shoes, carrying his swagger cane; and I straightened my shoulders and step out in cadence.

Looking back at my sporting days I was never a lover of long walks! However, my physical activities included cycling, skipping, swimming, light weights and lots of rock and roll (dance) that kept me reasonably fit!

Today, there are a large number of people with good intentions who start out their long walks, but peter out after several weeks. They found the walks boring, they don't have the time, or it is too hot, or I really don't want to get up and walk today, etc. I've been guilty of the same thoughts!

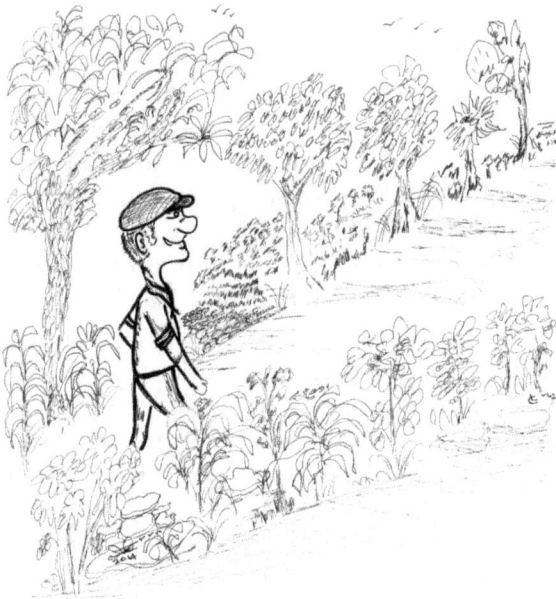

Walk, Observe and Draw

163

However, my short course circuit provides the answers to all the above excuses!

You may ask why the emphasis on this short course. The most important reason is that you pass your house after each circuit. You are motivated to do the walk, because you know that you can stop at any time. Yet, you will continue because you have set your goals and your own time limit. Nevertheless, this is not a torturous circuit, because it opens up opportunities for you to discover things and become creative.

When you start, observe the style of the houses, the design of the gardens, the floral arrangement in garden beds, the bushes and the types of trees that have been planted. After your 2nd circuit, notice for example, a tree trunk. Look at the bark, look at its texture, is it smooth or rough? Are there any designs that you notice? During your walk, visualize it, see it in your mind's eye, and now draw it in your mind. After completing your walk and are sitting down in the patio with your bottle of water, take pencil to paper and try to sketch what you have seen. Be creative!

It doesn't have to end here. During your walk consider the formation of clouds, see the different hues of a morning sunrise through the clouds or behind a hill, the mountain, and the trees; light up your eyes, your life and try your hand at water colour painting.

A starting palette, your paper, brush and water, and you are ready to open up a new world for yourself! For instance, commencing with several variegated washes, with blue at the top, and gradually changing from a yellow wash to green, towards the foreground. Paint in the mountains, and then the trees. You have your first watercolour. You have started a beautiful hobby that began with a 220 metre circuit from your front door.

Ask yourself! Do I really want to be a couch potato or do I want to add something new into my life. Do I look for self-pity or do I march to a new drumbeat to improve my lifestyle and health?

My walks are now becoming routine and I have another goal to add to the mix. It is the 24th January, 2013, and it is three months since my operation. To celebrate this wondrous occasion I have extended my circuit by doubling the length and walking the gentle hill! Ha! Thirty metres from the summit my knees began to sag, my shoulders drooped and I was puffing, I said to myself, 'It's OK you're 75! And you can catch your breath on the downhill walk.' now I walk it three times as part of my circuit. My friends "cheer me on."

I have successfully worked out my routine. I am up between 5.00am to 6.00am and have usually started my short course circuit by 6.00 o'clock or a little later. I am motivated and inspired by looking at each garden, of the vibrant colours of the flora, the growth of the plants. The ever-changing colours of the sky above; I am looking at the very life of nature itself, it is a spectacular picture of wonderment that I would not miss. Looking at nature's miracles, what more could you ask for in gaining your health and well-being and walking a 220 metre circuit right outside your front gate?

Yet, for us oldies our physical activity exercises need to cover four main areas: endurance, strength, flexibility and balance. You need to see your doctor and a physiotherapist to map out the ideal levels of a 30 minute activities program that will suit your needs in maintaining a good healthy lifestyle.

Although my reflux is dissipating gradually, at times I have had occasional twinges of tightness in the upper chest area. However, my previous stress test indicated that my heart was sound and I am advised that this tightness is probably due to tissue healing!

Since my heart operation in 2009, my left leg has been somewhat heavy in comparison to my right leg. It was the left leg that had the veins removed and relocated into the by-pass grafts. Since this recent operation, I have had nerve twinges occasionally in my left thigh and with a feeling of thickness on the soles of my feet. This is not related to gout! I hope that my circuit walking will alleviate this minor problem!

Chapter 6
Reflections

How sweet it is to be alive! To see another sunrise, to look at uncluttered, freshly mown lawns, delight in the vibrant hues of blue, yellow and red flowers nestled in well cared for garden beds and to marvel at the large variety of trees that stand as sentinels in each garden; to experience the joy, the laughter and experience life with loved ones, family and friends; the immeasurable experiences that life has to offer. Why wouldn't you want to be alive?

My wife Nela and I cannot express in words the deepest of gratitude to Dr Christina Steffen and her surgical team. They worked tirelessly in a 'touch and go' situation, so that this poor soul would see the break of dawn and to further enjoy the future journeys that life has in store for me!

To the hospital support teams, from the paramedics of the ambulance services, to a fantastic, wonderful group of Doctors and nurses who have woven a tradition of caring and kindness in helping patients regain their confidence towards a healthy physical recovery. I salute you.

Who could ask more from family and friends for their love and the need to see me back on my feet, doing the things I do best! What would we do without that wonderful, volunteer group of zany colleagues that inhabit the cardiac rehabilitation unit? Being former patients themselves and knowing the emotions that are deep within, they instill into cardiac patients the confidence and the realization that there is no room for self-pity or idleness. A meaningful life lies ahead of them after they complete their rehabilitation program. Those volunteers motivated me with their smiles, laughter and their well-wishes. Nine volunteers with some 45 or more combined years of volunteering in the Unit speaks highly of their worth to the Cardiac Rehabilitation Program. They are a family, they are my family!

Having been discharged on Saturday, 3rd November 2013, I was still weak, lacked energy and had little appetite. I knew that my home environment would give me more independence to fully work on my recovery. However, I did not fully realize the stress and strain that would be placed on Nela's shoulders during the caring stage of my rehabilitation as she had her own health problems to face.

I cannot recollect speaking to the hospital social worker during my nine day sojourn in the 'House that Health Built!' Although the ward nurse handling my discharge tried to contact the social worker, the Office was closed. We were given two telephone numbers to call on the following Monday, and that resulted in Caring Australia sending a representative to assess our needs.

Appointments, lengthy interviews and a large amount of paperwork later and Nela was classified as a carer. Ironically I had worked out my own schedule of rehabilitation exercises and my short, walking circuit. I wonder if the situation could have been improved through the initial contact with the social worker in the hospital!

Compared to the 'do's and don't' booklet, that I received after my 2009 heart operation; I was amazed that no such booklet or information sheet was forthcoming from the hospital upon my discharge for this latter operation. I had to flounder around searching for information over the internet to answer questions.

I have listed the following reflections that could be passed on to AAA patients on their discharge from hospital:

- The sooner you begin your rehabilitation exercises, the quicker will be your recovery. Walking the short circuit will give you confidence to regain your circulation and get your bowel movement back to normal. If you have swelling, this will begin to reduce. Associated lung problems will begin to clear up sooner. Healing of your battle scar is immensely improved.
- Persist in your breathing exercises. This will ensure the expansion of your lungs completely. These exercises may be uncomfortable at first, but they will clear any fluid that may be on your lungs.
- For many weeks after the operation, you will feel tired, but this will improve as you stride out in your walking activity.
- A week after you leave hospital, the rest of your stitches or staples will be removed by your own Doctor.
- If you have prolonged constipation or if diarrhoea persists, see your GP immediately. Dehydration will become a problem and so could reflux. A soft, bland diet for a few weeks will help and you

can move on to solid foods.

- No golf swings! Arm curls and shoulder raises with one kilo weights only, but again see your Doctor. Your rehabilitation will require endurance, flexibility, balance and physical activities that will increase as your recovery progresses.. Check with your surgeon if a rehabilitation program is available.

- Remember you are not a weight lifter! Your surgical operation needs to heal. Don't strain or lift anything heavier than 5kg or the weight of two telephone directories, for at least 12 weeks after your operation to be on the safe side. I am in my 6th week and I have some tightness around the sternum area. Don't rush! Stay cool!

- If you experience severe or uncomfortable pain, palpitations or dizziness Remember! Do not follow the old adage of, 'no pain, no gain.' For you it is, 'pain, no gain!' In the cardio rehab where there is pain we stop the exercises and the patient is reassessed by the cardio nurse or physio. If pain persists call 000 for an ambulance or see your Doctor.

- Take the pain medication as prescribed by your Doctor. If you have ill-effects see your Doctor.

- Nausea or persistent vomiting means a trip to the Doctor or to hospital emergency, otherwise you could be causing damage to your stomach. Likewise if you have a chest or wound infection, don't put it off or leave it too late. Seek help.

- Don't get behind the wheel of your car until you get the go-ahead from your Doctor. Your insurance will not be covered if you are in an accident.

- Doctors and Nurses must be aware and sensitive in what they say in front of their patients. Negative words could be misconstrued and may leave the patient more depressed.

I was under the impression that I would need a follow-up with my surgeon after the operation, but it seems that 'no news, is good news, 'and that my own doctor would over-see this part of my recovery. However, there is a possibility that I may have fallen through a crack and was overlooked for the review!

It is now 11th January 2015; I have revised my walk from 110 metres to 40 metres. I feel the shorter walk is more beneficial as it tends to make me walk faster rather than get into a stroll. After my walk I complete two sets of my six kettle bell exercises that include the swing, clean and press with each hand, squats, Russian twist and the overhead. Each exercise is a timed 30 seconds with a 30 second rest. Kettle bells come in different weights; I use a 7.5kg weight. Wall pushups and wall/ball squats.

I weighed and measured myself at the beginning, but will not do so until a year is completed. I believe constant checks do more damage to your self esteem and the seed of "I'm not losing much so why continue!" takes effect. I look for the subtle differences within my body. Wow! I'm getting a sexy butt and I must be losing something as I can tie my shoe laces with ease as my stomach does not get in the way, or when I inhale deeply I notice a change in my love handles; at the shopping mall I feel as if I am walking tall. However, like all exercises ensure you ask your Doctor first. Well, I've done it! It is April and I have just twisted my shoulder and tendernitis has decided to throw a spanner into my exercise regime. Shoulder problems unfortunately take more time to mend.

In conclusion, the subconscious mind is the habit forming mind; imprint healthy thoughts through your motivating mantra. Telling your mind repeatedly over and over again that you are sick is like a VCR recorder saying, "Hey Mind! My body is sick, and it must be true." do not get into the "What ifs..." or into the realms of "self-pity," Lose the negativity of your thoughts, "let go!" Clear your mind of poisonous thoughts, detox your mind. Learn to meditate, do your deep breathing and relaxation exercises that will help you before and after your operation. Success is up to you. Good luck.

REFERENCES

Chapter 2   National Heart Foundation of Australia 2007

Chapter 3   'Guide to Cholesterol Lowering' Pfitzer Australia Pty Ltd

Chapter 5   National Heart Foundation of Australia 2007

Chapter 10   www.health.qld.gov.au/townsville hospital

Chapter 12   Cardiac Surgery Guide Booklet, Townsville Hospital

Chapter 12   Death by Prescription' Ray D. Strand M.D. 2003

Chapter 14   National Heart Foundation of Australia, 2007

Chapter 26   Book of Ki: Co-coordinating Mind and Body in Daily
               Life, Koichi Tohei, c 1976

Chapter 28   Mother Teresa of Calcutta, "On Kindness,"
               (search quotes.com)

GLOSSARY

Allopurinol	To prevent gout
Amiodarone	Regulate heart rhythm
Angiogram	Takes a special x-ray of your arteries
Asprin	Prevents heart attacks and strokes
Arterial line	Monitors blood pressure and taking blood samples
Atorvastatin	Lowers cholesterol (Lipitor)
BP	Blood Pressure
Blood Tests	Measures level of substances in the blood
CABG	Coronary artery by-pass graft
Central venous line	Drug infusion/fluids/monitoring venous pressures
Colchicine	Treat acute attack of gout
Dr	Doctor
ECG	Reads the heart's electrical impulses (ultrasound)
Ferrous Sulfate	Prevent/treat anaemia
GP	General Practitioner
ICU	Intensive Care Unit
INR	International Normalized Ratio (Warfarin)

INR Test	Indicates how long blood takes to clot
Metoprolol	Belongs to a group of medcine called beta-blocker
Monounsaturated fats	Can also help lower blood cholesterol
Omeprazole	Treat reflux disease
Polyunsaturated fats	Helps lower blood cholesterol
Saturated fats	Raises blood cholesterol
TEDS	Thrombo and Embolic Deterrent Stockings
Trans fats	Raises blood cholesterol/decreases good HDL
Warfarin	Treat/prevent blood clots

Ode to the Volunteers

These are the ones who give so much
To soothe patient fears with a tender touch.
They arrive each week with a smile so dear,
To impart their knowledge and move heavy gear!

They come in all shapes and ages,
And give of their time without any wages.
Each has a talent they are willing to share,
With patients who know how much they care.

They come in all weather, shine or rain,
To keep cardiac rehab staff sane.
We are very lucky, there is no doubt,
For our volunteers we can't do without.

To each one we'd like to say
Thanks for putting sunshine in each day.

Printed in the USA
CPSIA information can be obtained
at www.ICGtesting.com
CBHW071359030724
11076CB00012B/121